CONTENTS

INTRODUCTION

If you've had your blood cholesterol level tested and been told that it is too high, you will need to make changes to your eating habits. That doesn't mean going on a starvation diet, it means eating more foods that will actively help reduce the amount of cholesterol in your blood, and limiting those that increase it. This book will explain how and why in the simplest way possible. It's not cranky and it's packed with delicious, nutritious recipes.

WHAT IS CHOLESTEROL?

Cholesterol is a naturally occurring, soft, waxy substance, made by the liver, not just in humans but in all animals. It is essential for life. It is a component of every cell in the body. It is vital for the functioning of the central nervous system as well as being used to make vitamin D and to make bile to process fatty foods.

HOW CAN YOU HAVE TOO MUCH?

Research now shows that if we eat a large proportion of saturated fat (see page 8) the liver uses it to make an excess of cholesterol. So, it is important to reduce your saturated fat intake if you wish to to reduce your blood cholesterol level. There are also a few foods that contain a particularly high proportion of cholesterol. These are egg yolks, prawns (shrimp), offal (kidneys, liver, etc.) and fish roes. There is some controversy as to what effect these have on blood cholesterol levels but it is recommended that egg yolks be limited to a maximum of three a week, including those used in cooking. In this book, you'll find egg whites are often used instead of whole eggs. I have avoided the other very high cholesterol foods too as they are not essential for a healthy diet. However, eating them occasionally should not affect your blood cholesterol level in the long term.

WHAT HAPPENS IF YOU HAVE EXCESS CHOLESTEROL IN YOUR BLOOD?

Well, you've heard of plaque on your teeth that, if allowed to build up, causes gum disease. Too much cholesterol causes a similar sort of silting-up in the small arteries which supply your heart with blood. If not kept in check, it can block the arteries, so preventing proper flow to the heart and increasing the risk of coronary heart disease.

THE DIFFERENT TYPES OF FAT

Fat not only makes other food more palatable, it is also an essential part of a healthy, balanced diet. It provides warmth and energy and ensures our immune system and muscles work properly. It keeps our skin soft and supple too. We need a certain amount to allow our bodies to absorb the fat-soluble vitamins A, D, E and K, and to provide essential fatty acids. The problem is, most people eat too much – especially saturated fats (see below). Fat naturally occurs in most foods, but particularly in milk, cheese, meat, fish, eggs, grains, nuts and seeds, so we don't need to add more by spreading butter thickly on bread, dabbing it all over cooked vegetables before we eat them or pouring lashings of cream on our puds.

ARE ALL FATS THE SAME?

When you think of fat, you probably think only of the white stuff round meat and slabs of butter, margarine and lard (shortening). But vegetable oils like corn, olive or sunflower are also fats, as are fish oils such as cod liver oil. They can, however, be divided into three main groups:

Saturated fats are mostly animal fats and solidify at room temperature. They are found in largest quantities in meat, dairy products and many margarines. Most plant products are low in saturated fats. The exceptions are hydrogenised vegetable oils and palm and coconut oil which are all from plants; they, too, solidify at room temperature and are high in saturated fat. Everyone is advised to cut down on saturated fats and if you have a high blood cholesterol level, you must reduce the amount in your diet or you may risk coronary heart disease.

Polyunsaturated fats come in two types: 'omega 6 fatty acid's, mainly found in vegetable and seed oils and in polyunsaturated margarines. These can help lower your blood cholesterol level but should only be used in moderation. The other type, 'omega 3 fatty acids', are found mainly in oily fish such as mackerel and tuna, and are thought to help protect against heart disease.

Monounsaturated fats are found in highest quantities in olive oil, avocados and rapeseed oil. They are not thought to have any effect on blood cholesterol levels. In Mediterranean countries where they have a high consumption of olive oil, there is a relatively low incidence of coronary heart disease. But obesity is a common problem in later life, so the message is to consume only small quantities.

WHICH FATS SHOULD YOU CHOOSE?

All the above fats have the same number of calories and so are equally fattening. Controversy still rages over the virtues of polyunsaturated versus monounsaturated fats. To reduce your blood cholesterol level, I recommend having very little saturated fat and a balance between polyunsaturated and monounsaturated fats; but, remember, you should not be having very much of any of them!

DAIRY PRODUCTS

Dairy products contain many things that are good for us: they are high in protein, and provide vitamins and minerals such as calcium for strong bones and teeth. It's their saturated fat content that you don't need, which is why you should stick to skimmed milk and the lowest-fat cheeses, yoghurts and creams you can find.

A word of warning about cream substitutes: I noticed, purely by accident, that one of the cream substitutes made with a mixture of vegetable fats and buttermilk had a higher saturated fat content than the reduced-fat real cream. So, as I can't stress too often, it is worth reading labels and comparing the nutritional information on the different brands which will tell you how much saturated, polyunsaturated and monounsaturated fat they each contain. Remember, too, that cream of any kind, even the reduced-fat type, should be eaten as a treat only.

Cultured buttermilk, which tastes rather like crème frâche, is a good alternative with no saturated fat.

WAYS TO HELP REDUCE BLOOD CHOLESTEROL LEVELS

These are all healthy eating suggestions – remember, taking regular exercise is also important.

- Change to polyunsaturated and monounsaturated fats and reduce the amount you eat overall. If you need to lose weight too, choose a reduced-fat sunflower or olive oil spread, suitable for baking as well as spreading (read the labels). Use any fat very sparingly.

- Eat plenty of fresh fruit and vegetables.

- Eat cereals high in soluble fibre, such as oats, barley and rye.

- Eat some oily fish every week, such as mackerel, herring, salmon, sardines, trout and tuna.

- Eat plenty of pulses (dried peas, beans and lentils).

- Most nuts and seeds like walnuts, pine nuts and sesame seeds (high in polyunsaturates) and almonds, pecans, hazelnuts and raw peanuts (high in monounsaturates) make a healthy snack. Avoid brazils and coconut, however, as they are high in saturated fat.

Avoid the following foods or keep them to a minimum:

- All fat on meat and skin on poultry.

- Full-cream milk and milk products.

- Egg yolks. Have no more than two or three a week, including those in cooking. Ideally, substitute two egg whites for one whole egg in baking.

- Prawns (shrimp), liver, kidneys and heart, fish roes (eat only occasionally).

- Fatty processed meats like sausages, canned meats like corned beef or spam. Eat cured meats like extra-lean bacon or ham in moderation only.

- Standard commercial chocolates, cakes, biscuits and ice creams.

- Brazil nuts and coconut.

A HEALTHY BALANCE

For good health you must eat foods from the five main food groups listed below every day.

Carbohydrates (for energy). There are two types. The first, complex carbohydrates, are found mainly in starchy foods like bread, pasta, rice, wholegrain cereals (including breakfast cereals but avoid those with added salt or sugar coatings) and potatoes. They are very important in your diet so eat plenty. The second type, simple carbohydrates, are sugars. They occur naturally in food in forms such as sucrose (a mixture of glucose and fructose) in fruit and lactose (a mixture of glucose and galactose) in milk. We don't need extra sugar. Not only does it pile on unwanted calories, it causes tooth decay. I prefer to use honey for sweetening when possible, as it is sweeter than sugar so you need less of it.

Proteins (for tissue growth and repair). Animal proteins are found mainly in lean meat (preferably white meat), fish, dairy products (choose low-fat varieties) and eggs (eat only two or three a week); vegetable proteins are found mainly in pulses (dried peas, beans and lentils) and manufactured vegetable proteins like soya, quorn and tofu (bean curd). Eat two to three small portions a day.

Vitamins and minerals (for general well-being). Different ones are found in all foods but the best sources are fruit and vegetables, preferably fresh but also frozen or canned in water with no salt or sugar added. Eat at least five portions of fruit and vegetables daily and include plenty of leafy greens.

Fats (for warmth and energy). As I have said, fats occur naturally in foods so adding more is unnecessary. Use polyunsaturated or monounsaturated fats for cooking and spreading, and only very sparingly.

Fibre (to aid digestion). We should all be eating more fibre. It consists of the cell walls of all parts of the plant – from the seeds, through to the roots, stems, leaves, flowers and fruit. It passes through the body, absorbing water and food waste products and helps to move the food through the gut to aid digestion. The best sources are wholegrain cereals, bread and pasta, brown rice, fruit and vegetables (including the skins where appropriate, e.g. on apples and potatoes), pulses, dried fruit and nuts, so eat plenty of all these. A high-fibre diet will help lower your blood cholesterol level. If you have had a low-fibre diet up until now, increase the fibre gradually. For example, have some white and some wholemeal bread, or a mixture of high- and low-fibre breakfast cereals, then gradually increase the amount of the high-fibre foods. If you drastically increase the fibre content too quickly, you may suffer from abdominal discomfort, flatulence and even diarrhoea while your body adjusts.

TOP TIPS TO REDUCE YOUR FAT INTAKE

- Grill (broil) or bake rather than fry (sauté).

- Brown meat by dry-frying in a non-stick pan, then spoon off any fat (reserving the juices).

- Use non-stick cookware or line tins (pans) with non-stick baking parchment rather than greasing them.

- Trim all fat off meat, use extra-lean cuts and remove skin from poultry.

- Choose canned fish in water rather than oil or brine.

- Don't add fat to vegetables before serving.

- Use sunflower or olive oil spread very sparingly on toast or bread – literally a scraping.

- Use skimmed milk instead of whole milk and the lowest-fat yoghurts and cheeses available (read the labels!).

FEEL THE DIFFERENCE IN JUST SEVEN DAYS

In this chapter I have put together a selection of recipes from this book to tempt your taste buds and get you used to the sort of meals you can enjoy using low-cholesterol menus. They are just a guide. In reality, for instance, you are not going to make all the bakes in one week; if you make a batch of Blueberry Muffins, you'll eat them up over a series of mornings, not have something different every day. And you won't make two cakes for tea. By the way, the teatime treats are exactly that. Only have snacks if you are hungry – they are most certainly not compulsory! A slice of cake or a home-made biscuit is ideal to round off dinner instead of one of the more formal puds too.

And a note about lunches. Sandwiches or filled rolls are an excellent choice. Use wholegrain breads, only a scraping of sunflower or olive oil spread, choose lean meat, chicken, fish like tuna or salmon (canned in water, preferably, or brine) or very low-fat cheese and lots of salad. If you must use mayonnaise, don't have too much and use a low-calorie variety.

DAY ONE

Breakfast	Glass of tomato juice Herrings in Oatmeal with wholemeal bread and butter (page 26) Tea or coffee with skimmed milk
Lunch	Cock-a-leekie Soup (page 37) Crusty bread Virtually fat-free fruit fromage frais
Teatime Snack	Granary Bread Stick (page 160)

Dinner	Lasagne al Forno (page 62)
	Dressed Green Salad (page 137)
	Mocha Mousse (page 153)

DAY TWO

Breakfast	Half a grapefruit
	Multi-cereal Cottage Loaf Rolls (page 24)
	with a scraping of sunflower or olive
	oil spread
	Reduced-sugar marmalade
	Tea or coffee with skimmed milk

Lunch	Mighty Chicken Loaf (page 64)
	English Mixed Salad (page 140)
	Apple

| *Teatime Snack* | Slice of Raspberry Angel Cake (page 170) |

| *Dinner* | Farmer's Beans (page 88) |
| | Tropical Fruit Salad (page 156) |

DAY THREE

Breakfast	Glass of pure orange juice
	Real Oatmeal Porridge (page 21)
	Tea or coffee with skimmed milk

Lunch	Haricot Bean and Ratatouille Soup
	(page 34) with crusty bread
	Apple

| *Teatime Snack* | Slice of Date and Walnut Loaf (page 172) |

Dinner	Chicken Shack Pie (page 60)
	Melon with Minted Raspberry
	Drizzle (page 157)

DAY FOUR

Breakfast	Glass of pure orange juice Blueberry Breakfast Muffins (page 22) Tea or coffee with skimmed milk
Lunch	Mozzarella-topped Aubergines (page 53) Garlic and Herb Bread (page 163) Orange
Teatime Snack	Almond Shortbread Slice (page 168)

Dinner	Kentucky Baked Turkey (page 82)
	Jacket-baked Potatoes with Yoghurt
	    and Chives (page 125)
	Peas and sweetcorn
	Rich and Creamy Brown Rice Pudding
	    (page 145)

DAY FIVE

Breakfast	Slice of melon Potato and Bacon Cakes (page 28) Tea or coffee with skimmed milk
Lunch	Soused Mackerel (page 106) with salad Virtually fat-free yoghurt with honey
Teatime Snack	Hazelnut Macaroon (page 169)
Dinner	Chicken Biryani (page 68) Green Pepper and Onion Salad (page 139) Honeyed Kiwis and Oranges (page 154)

DAY SIX

Breakfast	Glass of pure grapefruit juice Better-than-bought Muesli (page 20) Tea or coffee with skimmed milk
Lunch	Flageolet and Tuna Vinaigrette (page 55) A few strawberries and a virtually fat-free vanilla yoghurt
Teatime Snack	Poppy Seed Scone (page 166)

Dinner	Italian Crostini (page 48)
	Pork Medallions with Juniper and
	    Port (page 90)
	Savoury Potato Cake (page 124)
	Broccoli
	Profiteroles with Hot Chocolate
	    Sauce (page 148)

DAY SEVEN

Breakfast	Glass of pure orange juice The Lean English Breakfast (page 30) Tea or coffee with skimmed milk

Lunch	Pot Roast Paprika Chicken with Rice
	    (page 70)
	Spotted Dick (page 144) with Low-fat
	    Custard (page 180)

Teatime Snack	Slice of Chocolate Angel Cake Deluxe (page 171)
Dinner	Golden Root Soup (page 40) Crusty bread Banana

NOTES ON THE RECIPES

- All spoon measures are level: 1 tsp = 5 ml
                                        1 tbsp = 15 ml.

- Ingredients are given in metric, imperial and American measures. Use only one set per recipe, never a combination.

- Eggs are medium unless otherwise stated.

- If you choose a low-fat spread, make sure it is suitable for baking and frying (read the labels).

- All herbs are fresh unless dried are specifically called for. If substituting dried, use only half the quantity or less as they are very pungent, but chopped, frozen varieties are a better substitute than dried.

- Always wash, dry, peel and core, if necessary, any fresh produce before use. Only peel produce if really necessary as the outer layers contain valuable fibre.

- All preparation and cooking times are approximate and are intended as a guide only.

- Always preheat the oven unless it is fan-assisted and cook on the centre shelf unless otherwise stated.

- The saturated fat, cholesterol and fibre contents indicated refer to the individual recipe only and do not include any serving suggestions.

COMPLETE BREAKFASTS

Breakfast is probably the most important meal of the day. You need to refuel first thing to be sure that your body functions at its best during the morning. There is every type of sustenance here – for the cereal and toasties, for lovers of the hearty cooked breakfast and even for the I-can't-really-face-it brigade! In each case allow yourself a small glass of pure fruit juice or a piece of fresh fruit as well (the vitamin C helps your body absorb the iron in the cereal), plus a cup of tea or coffee, either black or with skimmed milk.

Better-than-bought Muesli

SERVES 8–10

★ VERY LOW SATURATED FAT ★ VERY LOW CHOLESTEROL ★ HIGH FIBRE

175 g/6 oz/1½ cups rolled oats

25 g/1 oz/½ cup wheat bran

25 g/1 oz/¼ cup sesame seeds

25 g/1 oz/¼ cup chopped hazelnuts

50 g/2 oz/⅓ cup raisins

50 g/2 oz/⅓ cup sultanas (golden raisins)

50 g/2 oz/⅓ cup ready-to-eat prunes, stoned (pitted) and chopped

50 g/2 oz/⅓ cup dried banana slices

A good pinch of ground cinnamon

Skimmed milk, to serve

1 Mix the oats and bran in a bowl.

2 Toast the sesame seeds and hazelnuts under the grill (broiler) or in a frying pan (skillet), turning to prevent burning.

3 Add to the bowl with the remaining ingredients. Mix well. Store in an airtight container. Serve with enough skimmed milk to moisten.

Real Oatmeal Porridge

SERVES 4

✴ VERY LOW SATURATED FAT ✴ VERY LOW CHOLESTEROL ✴ HIGH FIBRE

You can, of course make quick porridge with rolled oats, but this creamy concoction is far superior.

1.2 litres/2 pts/5 cups water

150 g/5 oz/1⅓ cups medium oatmeal

1.5 ml/¼ tsp salt

Skimmed milk and clear honey, to serve

1 Put the water in a heavy-based saucepan and bring to the boil.

2 Add the oatmeal in a steady stream, stirring all the time.

3 Bring back to the boil, turn the heat down as low as possible, cover and simmer very gently for 10 minutes, stirring occasionally.

4 Add the salt, stir again, cover and simmer very gently for a further 10–15 minutes, stirring occasionally until smooth and creamy.

5 Spoon into bowls, add skimmed milk and drizzle a little honey over the surface.

Blueberry Breakfast Muffins

MAKES 16–18

★ LOW SATURATED FAT ★ LOW CHOLESTEROL ★ HIGH FIBRE

300 ml/½ pt/1¼ cups boiling water

75 g/3 oz/½ cup dried blueberries

40 g/1½ oz/3 tbsp sunflower or olive oil spread

60 ml/4 tbsp clear honey

*225 g/8 oz/2 cups self-raising (self-rising)
wholemeal flour*

5 ml/1 tsp baking powder

Finely grated rind of ½ lemon

A pinch of grated nutmeg

1 egg, beaten

1 Mix the water with the blueberries and sunflower or olive oil spread and leave to soak, cooling, until the mixture is just warm.

2 Stir in the remaining ingredients.

3 Turn into the sections of tartlet tins (patty pans), lined with paper cake cases (cup cake papers), and bake in a preheated oven at 180°C/350°F/gas mark 4 for about 20 minutes until risen and the centres spring back when pressed.

4 Transfer to a wire rack to cool. Store in an airtight container. Serve warm or cold.

Carroty Yoghurt Muffins

★ VERY LOW SATURATED FAT ★ VERY LOW CHOLESTEROL ★ HIGH FIBRE

2 large carrots, grated

90 ml/6 tbsp clear honey

100 g/4 oz/1 cup wholemeal flour

225 g/8 oz/2 cups oat bran

5 ml/1 tsp baking powder

2.5 ml/½ tsp bicarbonate of soda (baking soda)

50 g/2 oz/½ cup walnuts, finely chopped

75 g/3 oz/½ cup raisins

2.5 ml/½ tsp mixed (apple-pie) spice

30 ml/2 tbsp sunflower oil

120 ml/4 fl oz/½ cup low-fat plain yoghurt

250 ml/8 fl oz/1 cup skimmed milk

2 egg whites

1 Line 16 sections of tartlet tins (patty pans) with paper cake cases (cup cake papers).

2 Mix all the ingredients together thoroughly.

3 Spoon into the cases and bake in a preheated oven at 200°C/400°F/gas mark 6 for about 20 minutes until risen and the centres spring back when pressed. Cool on a wire rack.

Multi-cereal Cottage Loaf Rolls

MAKES 6

★ VERY LOW SATURATED FAT ★ VERY LOW CHOLESTEROL ★ HIGH FIBRE

225 g/8 oz/2 cups strong plain (bread) flour

75 g/3 oz/¾ cup wholemeal flour

75 g/3 oz/¾ cup barley or rye flour

50 g/2 oz/½ cup oat bran

2.5 ml/½ tsp salt

10 ml/2 tsp easy-blend dried yeast

15 ml/1 tbsp olive oil

15 ml/1 tbsp clear honey

300 ml/½ pt/1¼ cups hot water

90 ml/6 tbsp low-fat fromage frais and a little reduced-sugar cherry jam (conserve), to serve

1 Mix the flours together in a bowl with the oat bran. Stir in the salt and yeast.

2 Blend the olive oil, honey and water together and mix to form a firm dough.

3 Knead well on a lightly floured surface until smooth and elastic.

4 Return to the bowl, cover with a damp cloth and leave in a warm place for about 1 hour until doubled in bulk.

5 Re-knead, then divide the dough into six equal pieces. Take a third off each piece and roll into a ball. Roll the larger pieces into balls.

6 Place the larger pieces well apart on a non-stick baking (cookie) sheet, dusted with flour. Top each with a smaller ball and then, using a floured finger, plunge down through the small ball into the larger ball to form the traditional cottage loaf shape.

7 Leave in a warm place for about 30 minutes until doubled in size. Bake in a preheated oven at 230°C/450°F/gas mark 8 for about 15 minutes until risen, golden and the bases sound hollow when tapped.

8 Cool on a wire rack. Serve warm or cold with fromage frais and cherry jam.

Herrings in Oatmeal

★ VERY LOW SATURATED FAT ★ LOW CHOLESTEROL ★ HIGH FIBRE

Use mackerel if you prefer.

4 even-sized herrings, cleaned and heads removed

Freshly ground black pepper

10 ml/2 tsp lemon juice

50–75 g/2–3 oz/½–¾ cup medium oatmeal

30 ml/2 tbsp chopped parsley

Lemon wedges and sprigs of parsley, to garnish

4 thin slices of wholemeal bread, spread with a scraping of sunflower or olive oil spread and cut into triangles, to serve

1 Split the herrings along the stomach and open out flat, skin-sides up. Run your thumb firmly up and down the backbone of each to loosen. Lift out the back bones and remove as many loose bones as possible.

2 Season thoroughly with freshly ground black pepper and sprinkle with lemon juice.

3 Mix the oatmeal and parsley together in a shallow dish. Press the fish into the oatmeal on both sides, to coat thoroughly.

4 Heat a non-stick frying pan (skillet). Cook the fish, one or two at a time, skin-sides up first, for about 3–4 minutes on each side until golden and cooked through. Keep the first ones warm in a low oven while cooking the remainder. Garnish with lemon wedges and parsley sprigs before serving with the triangles of bread and spread.

Salmon Kedgeree

SERVES 4

✴ VERY LOW SATURATED FAT ✴ LOW CHOLESTEROL ✴ HIGH FIBRE

175 g/6 oz/¾ cup brown long-grain rice

50 g/2 oz peas, frozen or fresh, shelled

175 g/6 oz salmon tail fillet, skinned

5 ml/1 tsp curry powder

60 ml/4 tbsp skimmed milk

30 ml/2 tbsp chopped parsley

A pinch of salt

Freshly ground black pepper

2 tomatoes, cut into neat chunks

5 ml/1 tsp lemon juice

Lemon wedges, to garnish

1 Cook the rice in plenty of boiling water for about 30 minutes or until tender. Add the peas after 25 minutes. Drain and return to the pan.

2 Meanwhile, dust the fish with the curry powder and place in a shallow pan with the milk. Cover and cook gently for 6–8 minutes until just tender and the fish flakes easily with a fork.

3 Break the fish into neat pieces.

4 Add the fish and its cooking liquid to the cooked rice with half the parsley, the salt and lots of pepper, the tomatoes and lemon juice. Toss over a gentle heat until piping hot. Pile on to hot plates, sprinkle with the remaining parsley and garnish with lemon wedges before serving.

Potato and Bacon Cakes

SERVES 4–6

★ VERY LOW SATURATED FAT ★ VERY LOW CHOLESTEROL ★ HIGH FIBRE

This is a delicious way of having a little bacon for a treat.

450 g/1 lb potatoes

25 g/1 oz/2 tbsp sunflower or olive oil spread

50 g/2 oz/½ cup wholemeal flour

**2 rashers (slices) of extra-lean, reduced-salt, unsmoked
back bacon, rinded and diced**

15 ml/1 tbsp snipped chives

15 ml/1 tbsp caraway seeds

3 tomatoes, each cut into 4 slices

1　Peel and cut the potatoes into even-sized pieces. Boil in water until tender.

2　Drain and mash with the spread, then beat in the flour.

3　Meanwhile, dry-fry the bacon in a non-stick frying pan (skillet) until cooked through. Drain on kitchen paper (paper towels). Add to the potato mixture with the chives and mix well. Wipe out the pan to clean it thoroughly.

4　Shape into 12 cakes and flatten slightly, pressing a few caraway seeds into the surface of each.

5　Heat the frying pan thoroughly, then cook the rounds for 3 minutes on each side until golden brown and slightly puffy.

6　Meanwhile, place the tomato slices on a flameproof plate and warm briefly under the grill (broiler).

7　Top each potato cake with a slice of tomato before serving.

The Good Morning Breakfast in a Glass

SERVES 1

★ VERY LOW SATURATED FAT ★ VERY LOW CHOLESTEROL ★ HIGH FIBRE

1 ripe banana

100 ml/3½ fl oz/6½ tbsp skimmed milk

125 g/4½ oz/1 small carton low-fat vanilla yoghurt

15 ml/1 tbsp oat bran

1 Peel the banana, break into small pieces and place in a blender or food processor.

2 Add a little of the milk and process until smooth.

3 Add the remaining ingredients and run the machine until thick and frothy.

4 Pour into a glass and serve.

The Lean English Breakfast

SERVES 4

★ LOW SATURATED FAT ★ FAIRLY LOW CHOLESTEROL ★ SOME FIBRE

Have this no more than once a week

4 rashers (slices) of extra-lean back bacon, rinded

2 tomatoes, halved

Freshly ground black pepper

25 g/1 oz/2 tbsp sunflower or olive oil spread

2 slices of bread

100 g/4 oz button mushrooms

30 ml/2 tbsp water

2 whole eggs

4 egg whites

45 ml/3 tbsp skimmed milk

A pinch of salt

1 Put the bacon and halved tomatoes under the grill (broiler). Sprinkle the tomatoes with pepper. Spread half the sunflower or olive oil spread on both sides of the bread. Cut into halves and lay on the grill rack. Grill (broil) until cooked to your liking, turning once. Remove foods as they are cooked and keep warm.

2 Meanwhile, put the mushrooms in a saucepan with the water and season with pepper. Cover and cook gently for 5 minutes until tender.

3 Melt the remaining spread in a non-stick saucepan. Whisk in the eggs and egg whites together with the milk and salt. Add a good grinding of pepper. Cook over a gentle heat, stirring all the time until scrambled. Do not allow to boil.

4 Arrange all the items on warm plates and serve.

Tomato Wakener

SERVES 1

★ ALMOST NO SATURATED FAT ★ VERY LOW CHOLESTEROL ★ LOW FIBRE

3 ripe tomatoes, quartered

60 ml/4 tbsp pure orange juice

A good pinch of chilli powder

A dash of soy sauce

Freshly ground black pepper

30 ml/2 tbsp low-fat fromage frais

Ice cubes

1 Purée the tomatoes in a blender or food processor.

2 Add the remaining ingredients and blend again.

3 Pour over ice cubes in a tall glass and drink straight away.

Mango Smoothie

SERVES 2

★ VERY LOW SATURATED FAT ★ VERY LOW CHOLESTEROL ★ SOME FIBRE

1 small ripe mango

1 banana

120 ml/4 fl oz/1 cup pineapple juice

*170 g/6½ oz/1 small can of low-fat
evaporated milk, well chilled*

Lemon juice, to taste

1 Peel the mango, cut all the flesh off the stone (pit) and place in a blender or food processor. Peel the banana, break into pieces and add.

2 Add half the pineapple juice and purée until smooth. Blend in the remaining juice.

3 Meanwhile, whisk the evaporated milk until thick and doubled in bulk. Whisk in the fruit mixture. Sharpen with lemon juice. Pour into glasses and serve.

SOUPS FOR EVERY OCCASION

Soups make delicious, simple and nutritious lunches or suppers, served with crusty bread. They can also be served (in smaller portions) as starters before a light main course. Flavours often improve if the soup is made one day and then reheated (until piping hot!) the next. If you are doing this, always cover the freshly cooked soup while it cools and as soon as it's cold, store it in the fridge.

Haricot Bean and Ratatouille Soup

★ VERY LOW SATURATED FAT ★ NO CHOLESTEROL ★ HIGH FIBRE

1 onion, finely chopped

1 garlic clove, crushed

15 ml/1 tbsp olive oil

1 aubergine (eggplant), diced

1 red (bell) pepper, diced

1 green pepper, diced

1 courgette (zucchini), diced

425 g/15 oz/1 large can of haricot (navy) beans, drained and thoroughly rinsed

400 g/14 oz/1 large can of chopped tomatoes

1 vegetable stock cube

15 ml/1 tbsp tomato purée (paste)

2.5 ml/½ tsp dried mixed herbs

A pinch of salt

Freshly ground black pepper

1 Fry (sauté) the onion and garlic in the oil in a large saucepan for 2 minutes, stirring.

2 Add all the remaining ingredients. Fill the tomato can with water and add to the pan. Repeat with a further canful of water.

3 Bring to the boil, reduce the heat, part-cover and simmer for 30 minutes until really tender. Ladle into warm soup bowls and serve.

Danish Pea Soup

SERVES 6

★ VERY LOW SATURATED FAT ★ VERY LOW CHOLESTEROL ★ HIGH FIBRE

75 g/3 oz/½ cup yellow split peas

75 g/3 oz/scant ½ cup pearl barley

15 ml/1 tbsp olive oil

1 large onion, finely chopped

*1.2 litres/2 pts/5 cups vegetable or chicken stock,
made with 2 stock cubes*

30 ml/2 tbsp tomato purée (paste)

Freshly ground black pepper

150 ml/¼ pt/⅔ cup skimmed milk

15 ml/1 tbsp snipped chives

15 ml/1 tbsp chopped parsley, to garnish

1 Soak the peas and barley in cold water overnight.
Drain.

2 Heat the oil in a saucepan and cook the onion gently,
stirring, for 3 minutes until softened but not browned.
Add the stock, peas and barley. Bring to the boil, skim
the surface, part-cover and simmer gently for 1½ hours.

3 Purée in a blender or food processor with the tomato
purée. Return to the saucepan and add pepper to taste.

4 Stir in the milk and chives and heat through.

5 Ladle into warm bowls and sprinkle with chopped
parsley before serving.

Rich Mushroom Soup

SERVES 6

★ VERY LOW SATURATED FAT ★ VERY LOW CHOLESTEROL ★ LOW FIBRE

1 small onion, chopped

350 g/12 oz button mushrooms, roughly chopped

15 g/½ oz/1 tbsp sunflower or olive oil spread

*150 ml/¼ pt/⅔ cup chicken or vegetable stock,
made with ½ stock cube*

30 ml/2 tbsp plain (all-purpose) flour

450 ml/¾ pt/2 cups skimmed milk

A pinch of salt

Freshly ground black pepper

30 ml/2 tbsp finely chopped parsley

30 ml/2 tbsp low-fat fromage frais

1 Cook the onion and mushrooms gently in the spread for 3 minutes, stirring, until softened but not browned.

2 Add the stock, stir, cover, reduce the heat to low and simmer gently for 10 minutes, stirring occasionally, until tender.

3 Blend the flour with a little of the milk. Stir into the mushrooms with the remaining milk.

4 Bring to the boil and cook for 2 minutes, stirring.

5 Purée in a blender or food processor and return to the saucepan. Season, then stir in the parsley and fromage frais. Reheat but do not boil.

6 Ladle into warm soup bowls and serve.

Cock-a-leekie Soup

SERVES 6

★ LOW SATURATED FAT ★ LOW CHOLESTEROL ★ HIGH FIBRE

2 large leeks, thinly sliced

2 chicken portions, skin removed

75 g/3 oz/scant ½ cup pearl barley

1 bouquet garni sachet

1.75 litres/3 pts/7½ cups chicken stock, made with 3 stock cubes

A pinch of salt

Freshly ground black pepper

8 prunes, quartered and stoned (pitted)

30 ml/2 tbsp chopped parsley

1 Put all the ingredients except the prunes and parsley in a large saucepan.

2 Bring to the boil, reduce the heat, part-cover and simmer gently for 1 hour. Add the prunes and cook for a further 30 minutes until the barley and chicken are tender.

3 Lift the chicken out of the soup. Take all the meat off the bones and cut into small pieces.

4 Return to the pan and simmer for a further 5 minutes. Taste and re-season, if necessary. Discard the bouquet garni. Stir in the parsley and serve.

Chilled Guacamole Soup

★ VERY LOW SATURATED FAT ★ VERY LOW CHOLESTEROL ★ SOME FIBRE

2 large ripe avocados

1 shallot, grated

15 ml/1 tbsp lemon juice

15 ml/1 tbsp olive oil

10 ml/2 tsp Worcestershire sauce

1.5 ml/¼ tsp Tabasco sauce

*300 ml/½ pt/1¼ cups vegetable stock, made with
1 stock cube and cooled*

450 ml/¾ pt/2 cups skimmed milk

5 cm/2 in piece of cucumber, very finely chopped

2 tomatoes, finely chopped

Freshly ground black pepper

30 ml/2 tbsp snipped chives, to garnish

1 Peel the avocados, remove the stones (pits) and place in a blender or food processor with the shallot, lemon juice and oil. Run the machine until smooth.

2 Add the Worcestershire and Tabasco sauces and the cooled stock. Run the machine again.

3 Turn the mixture into a bowl and stir in the remaining ingredients. Chill until ready to serve.

4 Ladle into soup bowls and sprinkle each with snipped chives before serving.

Flageolet and Almond Soup

★ VERY LOW SATURATED FAT ★ NO CHOLESTEROL ★ HIGH FIBRE

100 g/4 oz/1 cup dried green flageolet beans, soaked overnight in cold water

2 litres/3½ pts/8½ cups water

1 bunch of spring onions (scallions), finely chopped

1 garlic clove, crushed

15 ml/1 tbsp sunflower oil

2 celery sticks, finely chopped

2 vegetable stock cubes

100 g/4 oz/1 cup ground almonds

A pinch of salt

Freshly ground black pepper

30 ml/2 tbsp chopped parsley

30 ml/2 tbsp toasted flaked (slivered) almonds

1 Drain the beans and place in a saucepan. Add 1 litre/1¾ pts/4¼ cups of the water. Bring to the boil and boil rapidly for 10 minutes. Part-cover and simmer gently for about 1 hour or until the beans are tender.

2 Add all the remaining ingredients except the parsley and flaked almonds and simmer for 30 minutes.

3 Taste and re-season, if necessary.

4 Ladle into warm soup bowls and sprinkle with the parsley and flaked almonds before serving.

Golden Root Soup

✴ VERY LOW SATURATED FAT ✴ NO CHOLESTEROL ✴ HIGH FIBRE

1 onion, chopped

*15 g/½ oz/1 tbsp sunflower or olive oil spread,
plus a little for spreading*

½ small swede (rutabaga), diced

1 potato, diced

1 small parsnip, diced

1 large carrot, diced

½ small celeriac (celery root), diced

*1.5 litres/2½ pts/6 cups vegetable stock,
made with 2 stock cubes*

1 bay leaf

A pinch of salt

Freshly ground black pepper

2 slices of wholemeal bread

5 ml/1 tsp paprika

30 ml/2 tbsp chopped parsley

1 Fry (sauté) the onion in the measured quantity of spread for 2 minutes, stirring until softened but not browned.

2 Add the remaining vegetables, the stock, bay leaf, salt and a little pepper.

3 Bring to the boil, part-cover, reduce the heat and simmer for 30 minutes.

4 Remove the bay leaf and purée the mixture in a blender or food processor.

5 Return to the pan and re-season, if necessary. Heat through.

6 Meanwhile, spread the bread with a very thin scraping of sunflower or olive oil spread. Cut into small cubes. Dust with the paprika. Dry-fry in a frying pan (skillet), tossing until crisp and brown.

7 Ladle the soup into warm bowls. Sprinkle with the parsley before serving with the croûtons handed separately.

Chinese Mock Seaweed Soup

SERVES 4

✱ VERY LOW SATURATED FAT ✱ VERY LOW CHOLESTEROL ✱ HIGH FIBRE

225 g/8 oz curly kale

*1.2 litres/2 pts/5 cups chicken stock, made with
2 stock cubes*

1 bunch of spring onions (scallions), chopped

15 ml/1 tbsp sunflower oil

45 ml/3 tbsp reduced-salt soy sauce

1.5 ml/¼ tsp ground ginger

30 ml/2 tbsp sherry

Freshly ground black pepper

1 egg white

A pinch of salt

15 ml/1 tbsp snipped chives

1 Discard any thick stalks from the kale and shred.

2 Bring the stock to the boil, add the kale and cook for
   5 minutes.

3 Meanwhile, fry (sauté) the spring onions in the oil for
   3 minutes, stirring.

4 Add to the kale and the stock and simmer for a further
   30 minutes.

5 Purée in a blender or food processor. Return to the pan
   and stir in the soy sauce, a pinch of ginger, the sherry
   and lots of pepper. Reheat.

6   Whisk the egg white with the salt until stiff. Fold in the chives.

7   Ladle the soup into flameproof bowls and put a spoonful of the egg white on top of each.

8   Flash under a preheated grill (broiler) for about 2 minutes to brown and set the egg white. Serve straight away.

New-age Partan Bree

SERVES 6

★ VERY LOW SATURATED FAT ★ LOW CHOLESTEROL ★ HIGH FIBRE

50 g/2 oz/¼ cup brown long-grain rice

900 ml/1½ pts/3¾ cups water

2 chicken stock cubes

1 large cooked crab

90 ml/6 tbsp skimmed milk powder

5 ml/1 tsp anchovy essence (extract)

10 ml/2 tsp tomato purée (paste)

A pinch of salt

Freshly ground white pepper

10 ml/2 tsp cornflour (cornstarch)

30 ml/2 tbsp skimmed milk

150 ml/¼ pt/⅔ cup buttermilk or low-fat crème fraîche

15 ml/1 tbsp chopped parsley, to serve

1 Put the rice and water in a saucepan with the stock cubes. Bring to the boil, reduce the heat and simmer for about 40 minutes until the rice is tender, stirring occasionally.

2 Pick all the brown and white crab meat out of the body and small legs of the crab and place in a food processor or blender. Crack the large claws, remove the meat, cut into neat pieces and put to one side.

3 Pour the cooked rice and liquid into the blender or food processor with the brown and white meat from the body and small claws. Purée. Add the milk powder, anchovy essence and tomato purée and run the machine again until well blended.

4 Return to the saucepan. Season to taste. Blend the cornflour with the milk and stir in. Bring to the boil and cook for 1 minute, stirring. Stir in the buttermilk or crème fraîche and the claw meat. Taste and re-season, if necessary.

5 Ladle into warm bowls and sprinkle with the parsley before serving.

Clear Garlic Broth
with Noodles

SERVES 4

★ VERY LOW SATURATED FAT ★ ALMOST NO CHOLESTEROL ★ SOME FIBRE

2 potatoes, scrubbed and chopped

2 carrots, scrubbed and chopped

2 outer celery sticks, chopped, including any leaves

1 large onion, chopped

1 small bay leaf

Salt and freshly ground black pepper

1.5 litres/2½ pts/6 cups water

1 bulb of garlic, separated into cloves and peeled

15 ml/1 tbsp olive oil

1 large sprig of fresh thyme

6 sage leaves

75 g/3 oz vermicelli, broken into small pieces

1 Put the potatoes, carrots, celery and onion in a large saucepan with the bay leaf, a little salt, lots of pepper and the water. Bring to the boil, part-cover, reduce the heat and simmer for 2 hours.

2 Strain the stock and return to the rinsed-out saucepan. Add the remaining ingredients except the vermicelli, bring back to the boil, part-cover, reduce the heat and simmer gently for 30 minutes.

3 Strain again, return to the heat and add the vermicelli. Simmer gently for about 5 minutes or until the pasta is tender. Taste and re-season, if necessary. Serve in colourful bowls with no garnish.

STARTERS AND LIGHT MEALS

All the following recipes make
delicious appetisers but are
equally suitable for light lunches
or suppers with, perhaps, some
crusty bread, rolls or a side salad,
where appropriate.

Italian Crostini

SERVES 4 OR 8

★ VERY LOW SATURATED FAT ★ NO CHOLESTEROL ★ SOME FIBRE

8 large diagonal slices from a ciabatta loaf

1 large garlic clove

175 g/6 oz button mushrooms, finely chopped

30 ml/2 tbsp olive oil

15 ml/1 tbsp dry vermouth

Freshly ground black pepper

50 g/2 oz/⅓ cup stoned (pitted) black olives

5 ml/1 tsp lemon juice

15 ml/1 tbsp chopped basil

1 Lay the slices of bread on a baking (cookie) sheet. Cut the garlic clove in half and rub over all the surfaces of the bread. Then crush the garlic and reserve.

2 Bake the bread in a preheated oven at 180°C/350°F/gas mark 4 for about 20 minutes until golden.

3 Meanwhile, put the crushed garlic in a saucepan with the mushrooms, half the olive oil and the vermouth. Add a good grinding of pepper. Cook gently, stirring occasionally, for 5 minutes until soft.

4 Meanwhile, purée the olives with the remaining oil in a blender or food processor, stopping the machine and scraping down the sides, if necessary. Sharpen with the lemon juice.

5 Remove the bread from the oven. Spread with the olive paste and top with the chopped mushrooms. Sprinkle with the basil and serve straight away.

Smoked Mackerel with Watercress and Orange

SERVES 6

✱ VERY LOW SATURATED FAT ✱ LOW CHOLESTEROL ✱ SOME FIBRE

1 bunch of watercress

2 oranges

15 ml/1 tbsp olive oil

15 ml/1 tbsp pure orange juice

10 ml/2 tsp lemon juice

Freshly ground black pepper

5 ml/1 tsp horseradish relish

6 cooked smoked mackerel fillets

1 Trim the feathery stalks off the watercress and separate into sprigs. Place in a bowl.

2 Hold each orange over the bowl and cut off all the rind and pith. Cut the orange into segments and add to the bowl. Squeeze the membranes to extract any juice, then discard.

3 Whisk together the oil, orange and lemon juice, lots of pepper and the horseradish.

4 Pour over the watercress and orange and toss gently.

5 Lay the mackerel fillets on serving plates and arrange the salad to one side of each.

Asparagus with Walnut Vinaigrette

SERVES 6

★ VERY LOW SATURATED FAT ★ NO CHOLESTEROL ★ HIGH FIBRE

750 g/1½ lb thin asparagus spears

A pinch of salt

75 ml/5 tbsp white wine vinegar

30 ml/2 tbsp sunflower oil

15 ml/1 tbsp walnut oil

30 ml/2 tbsp water

50 g/2 oz/½ cup walnut pieces

A pinch of salt

Freshly ground black pepper

2.5 ml/½ tsp caster (superfine) sugar

15 ml/1 tbsp chopped tarragon

15 ml/1 tbsp chopped parsley

1 Trim off any thick, woody ends of the asparagus and tie the spears in two bundles. Stand the bundles in a large pan of boiling water with a pinch of salt added.

2 Bring back to the boil, cover with a lid, or foil if the bunches are too tall. Simmer for 10 minutes. Drain (reserving the liquid for soup or stock, if liked). Rinse the asparagus with cold water, drain again and leave until completely cold. Chill.

3 Meanwhile, put the remaining ingredients in a blender or food processor and run the machine until the mixture is thick and creamy. Chill.

5   When ready to serve, lay the asparagus on serving plates. Whisk the dressing again and spoon across the stems. Serve cold.

〜

Poor Man's Caviare

SERVES 4

★ VERY LOW SATURATED FAT ★ NO CHOLESTEROL ★ SOME FIBRE

1 large aubergine (eggplant)

1 shallot, finely chopped

1 small garlic clove, crushed

2 ripe tomatoes, skinned and chopped

30–45 ml/2–3 tbsp olive oil

Lemon juice, to taste

A pinch of salt

Freshly ground black pepper

15 ml/1 tbsp chopped parsley, to garnish

Wholemeal toast, to serve

1   Grill (broil) the aubergine, turning occasionally, until the skin is blackened and the aubergine feels soft when squeezed.

2   Cool slightly, then cut in half and scoop out the flesh, chop finely, and place in a bowl. Discard the skin.

3   Add the shallot, garlic and tomatoes and mix well.

4   Beat in enough of the oil, a drop at a time, until the mixture is glistening but not runny.

5   Add lemon juice and seasoning to taste.

6   Spoon into small pots, sprinkle with chopped parsley and serve with wholemeal toast.

Champignons à la Grecque

SERVES 6

★ VERY LOW SATURATED FAT ★ NO CHOLESTEROL ★ SOME FIBRE

*1 bunch of spring onions (scallions), chopped,
reserving a little of the green for garnish*

1 garlic clove, crushed

30 ml/2 tbsp olive oil

300 ml/½ pt/1¼ cups red wine

A pinch of salt

Freshly ground black pepper

2.5 ml/½ tsp dried oregano

450 g/1 lb button mushrooms

400 g/14 oz/1 large can of chopped tomatoes

5 ml/1 tsp finely grated lemon rind

A pinch of caster (superfine) sugar

Round lettuce leaves

6 slices of lemon, to garnish

1 Put the spring onions in a large saucepan with the garlic and oil. Cook gently for 2 minutes, stirring.

2 Add all the remaining ingredients except the lettuce leaves. Bring to the boil, reduce the heat and simmer for 20 minutes until the mushrooms are cooked and bathed in sauce.

3 Leave until cold, then chill.

4 When ready to serve, line six bowls with lettuce leaves. Spoon in the mushroom mixture. Top each with a twist of lemon and a sprinkling of spring onion tops.

Mozzarella-topped Aubergines

SERVES 6

★ VERY LOW SATURATED FAT ★ VERY LOW CHOLESTEROL ★ SOME FIBRE

1 garlic clove, halved

2 large aubergines (eggplants), sliced

A pinch of salt

Freshly ground black pepper

300 ml/½ pt/1¼ cups passata (sieved tomatoes)

30 ml/2 tbsp tomato purée (paste)

5 ml/1 tsp dried basil

100 g/4 oz/1 cup low-fat Mozzarella cheese, grated

1 Rub around the sides and bases of six shallow individual ovenproof dishes with the cut garlic, then discard.

2 Cook the aubergine slices in boiling water for 5 minutes until just tender. Drain.

3 Arrange in the prepared dishes. Season with the salt and lots of pepper.

4 Whisk the passata with the tomato purée and basil.

5 Spoon over the aubergines.

6 Sprinkle with the cheese, then bake in a preheated oven at 200°C/400°F/gas mark 6 for 15 minutes until the cheese has melted and is bubbling. Serve hot.

Avocados with Tuna Salsa

★ VERY LOW SATURATED FAT ★ LOW CHOLESTEROL ★ SOME FIBRE

185 g/6½ oz/1 medium can of tuna in water, drained

2 ripe tomatoes, seeded and finely chopped

1 shallot, finely chopped

1 small green (bell) pepper, seeded and finely chopped

1 small green or red chilli, seeded and finely chopped

Freshly ground black pepper

A dash of Worcestershire sauce

3 ripe avocados

Lemon juice

1 black olive, stoned (pitted) and cut into 6 slices

6 tiny sprigs of parsley

1   Mash the tuna thoroughly in a bowl.

2   Mix in the tomatoes, shallot, pepper and chilli. Season with pepper and Worcestershire sauce.

3   Halve the avocados, remove the stones (pits) and peel off all the skin with your fingers rather than a knife to leave a smooth shape. Brush all over with lemon juice.

4   Spread the salsa out on six small serving plates. Lay an avocado half, rounded side up, on each.

5   Top each round with a slice of olive and place a tiny sprig of parsley in the centre of each slice.

Flageolet and Tuna Vinaigrette

SERVES 4

★ VERY LOW SATURATED FAT ★ VERY LOW CHOLESTEROL ★ HIGH FIBRE

*425 g/15 oz/1 large can of flageolet beans,
rinsed and drained*

185 g/6½ oz/1 medium can of tuna in water, drained

1 small onion, sliced and separated into rings

1 small green (bell) pepper, diced

1 garlic clove, crushed

30 ml/2 tbsp olive oil

15 ml/1 tbsp white wine vinegar

5 ml/1 tsp chopped thyme

A pinch of salt

Freshly ground black pepper

15 ml/1 tbsp chopped parsley

1 Put the beans in a bowl with the tuna, onion and pepper.

2 Whisk all the remaining ingredients except the parsley together. Pour over and toss gently.

3 Cover and chill for 1 hour to allow the flavours to develop.

4 Spoon on to small plates and sprinkle with chopped parsley.

Warm Scallop, Bacon and Apple Salad

SERVES 4

★ VERY LOW SATURATED FAT ★ LOW CHOLESTEROL ★ FAIRLY HIGH FIBRE

175 g/6 oz ready-prepared mixed salad leaves

4 cherry tomatoes, quartered

5 cm/2 in piece of cucumber, diced

1 small red onion, sliced thinly and separated into rings

15 ml/1 tbsp olive oil

1 small onion, finely chopped

2 rashers (slices) of extra-lean back bacon, cut into small pieces

1 small red eating (dessert) apple, cored and diced

175 g/6 oz queen scallops

60 ml/4 tbsp cider

15 ml/1 tbsp snipped chives

Freshly ground black pepper

30 ml/2 tbsp cider vinegar

15 ml/1 tbsp water

Chopped parsley, to garnish

1 Arrange the salad leaves on four plates. Scatter the tomatoes, cucumber and red onion rings over.

2 Heat the oil in a large frying pan (skillet). Add the chopped onion, bacon and apple and fry (sauté) for 1 minute.

3 Add the scallops and cook, stirring, for 2–3 minutes.

4 Add the cider, chives and pepper and simmer for 2 minutes.

5 Lift the scallop and bacon mixture out of the pan with a draining spoon and place on the salad. Quickly add the vinegar, water and another good grinding of pepper to the juices and bring just to the boil. Spoon over the salads and sprinkle with chopped parsley before serving straight away.

Minted Melon with Garlic Cheese Bread

SERVES 6

★ VERY LOW SATURATED FAT ★ VERY LOW CHOLESTEROL ★ HIGH FIBRE

1 honeydew melon

30 ml/2 tbsp chopped mint

90 ml/6 tbsp apple juice

1 small wholemeal French stick

25 g/1 oz/2 tbsp sunflower or olive oil spread

75 g/3 oz/⅓ cup low-fat garlic and herb soft cheese

30 ml/2 tbsp chopped parsley

Freshly ground black pepper

A few small sprigs of mint, to garnish

1 Halve the melon and remove the seeds. Use a melon baller to scoop the flesh out of the shell, or peel and cut the fruit into dice.

2 Place in a sealable container and add the mint and apple juice. Cover and chill.

3 Cut the French stick into 12 slices, not quite through the base crust. Mash the spread with the cheese, parsley and lots of pepper. Spread between the slices.

4 Wrap in foil, shiny side in. Bake in a preheated oven at 200°C/400°F/gas mark 6 for 15 minutes until the crust feels crisp when squeezed.

5 Spoon the melon and juice into six small glass bowls and garnish each with small sprigs of mint. Serve with the hot garlic bread.

MEAT AND POULTRY
MAIN COURSES

I have chosen mostly poultry dishes for this section as they are naturally lower in fat, but there are also recipes that use the leaner cuts of pork, beef and lamb. If, however, you crave a slab of red meat, choose a small fillet steak, or a pork or lamb leg steak, trimmed of all fat. Brush with the minimum of olive or sunflower oil, season with freshly ground black pepper and grill (broil) rather than fry. Incidentally, you can substitute turkey for chicken and vice versa.

Chicken Shack Pie

SERVES 4

✴ LOW SATURATED FAT ✴ LOW CHOLESTEROL ✴ SOME FIBRE

This is a delicious low-fat version of cottage pie.

1 onion, finely chopped

350 g/12 oz extra-lean minced (ground) chicken

1 large carrot, grated

1 turnip, grated

75 g/3 oz frozen peas

**450 ml/¾ pt/2 cups chicken stock, made with
1 stock cube**

2.5 ml/½ tsp dried mixed herbs

Freshly ground black pepper

**750 g/1½ lb potatoes, peeled and cut into
even-sized pieces**

45 ml/3 tbsp skimmed milk

15 g/½ oz/1 tbsp sunflower or olive oil spread

5 ml/1 tsp Worcestershire sauce

30 ml/2 tbsp plain (all-purpose) flour

45 ml/3 tbsp cold water

2.5 ml/½ tsp paprika

Caraway Cabbage (see page 135), to serve

1 Put the onion and minced chicken in a large non-stick saucepan. Cook, stirring, for 5 minutes until the meat is browned and all the grains are separate. Spoon off any fat, but not the juices.

2 Add the carrot, turnip, peas and stock. Stir in the herbs and lots of pepper. Bring to the boil, stirring occasionally, reduce the heat, part-cover and simmer very gently for 20 minutes.

3 Meanwhile, cook the potatoes in boiling water until tender. Drain and mash with the milk, sunflower or olive oil spread and Worcestershire sauce.

4 Blend the flour with the water and stir into the chicken mixture. Bring to the boil and cook for 2 minutes, stirring until thickened.

5 Turn into an ovenproof dish. Spoon the potato on top and make rough patterns with a fork. Dust with paprika. Bake in a preheated oven at 200°C/400°F/gas mark 6 for 25 minutes until turning golden on top. Serve with Caraway Cabbage.

Lasagne al Forno

SERVES 4

⭑ LOW SATURATED FAT ⭑ LOW CHOLESTEROL ⭑ FAIRLY HIGH FIBRE

1 large onion, finely chopped

1 garlic clove, crushed

350 g/12 oz extra-lean minced (ground) turkey

1 carrot, finely chopped

75 g/3 oz button mushrooms, sliced

400 g/14 oz/1 large can of chopped tomatoes

30 ml/2 tbsp dry white vermouth (optional)

15 ml/1 tbsp tomato purée (paste)

2.5 ml/½ tsp dried oregano

A pinch of salt

Freshly ground black pepper

6 sheets of no-need-to-precook wholewheat lasagne

1 quantity of Cheese Sauce (see page 176)

Dressed Green Salad (see page 137)

---

1 Put the onion, garlic, turkey and carrot in a large non-stick saucepan. Cook, stirring, for 5 minutes until the meat is browned and all the grains are separate.

2 Add the mushrooms, tomatoes, vermouth, if using, the tomato purée, oregano, salt and lots of pepper. Bring to the boil, stirring, then reduce the heat and simmer for 15 minutes, stirring occasionally, until the meat is bathed in a rich sauce.

3 Spoon a little of the meat sauce in the base of a fairly shallow ovenproof dish. Top with a layer of lasagne, breaking it to fit. Layer the meat and lasagne in the dish, finishing with a layer of lasagne.

4 Spoon the cheese sauce over. Bake in a preheated oven at 190°C/375°F/gas mark 5 for 40 minutes until cooked through and golden on top. Serve hot with a Dressed Green Salad.

Mighty Chicken Loaf

SERVES 4

★ LOW SATURATED FAT ★ LOW CHOLESTEROL ★ FAIRLY HIGH FIBRE

1 onion, quartered

225 g/8 oz/2 cups cooked chicken, roughly cut up

2 slices of extra-lean cooked ham

25 g/1 oz/2 tbsp sunflower or olive oil spread

30 ml/2 tbsp browned breadcrumbs

100 g/4 oz button mushrooms, chopped

2.5 ml/½ tsp dried mixed herbs

90 ml/6 tbsp oat bran

1 Weetabix, crushed

150 ml/¼ pt/⅔ cup skimmed milk

1 egg, beaten

A pinch of salt

Freshly ground black pepper

300 ml/½ pt/1¼ cups passata (sieved tomatoes)

2.5 ml/½ tsp dried basil

*Seeded Roast Potatoes (see page 128) and a
mixed salad, to serve*

1 Mince (grind) the onion, chicken and ham or chop, not too finely, in a food processor.

2 Use a little of the spread to lightly grease a 450 g/ 1 lb loaf tin (pan). Coat with the breadcrumbs.

3 Melt the remaining spread in a saucepan. Add the mushrooms and herbs and fry (sauté) for 2 minutes, stirring. Sprinkle the oat bran over and stir for 1 minute. Add the Weetabix, milk and egg, then stir in the chicken mixture and season with the salt and some pepper.

4 Turn into the prepared tin and smooth the surface. Cover with foil and stand the tin in a roasting tin containing 2.5 cm/1 in boiling water. Bake in a preheated oven at 180°C/350°F/gas mark 4 for 1 hour, then remove the foil and cook for a further 30 minutes until firm and cooked through.

5 Meanwhile, warm the passata with the basil and a good grinding of pepper. Turn the loaf out on to a warm serving dish and serve sliced with the warm passata, Seeded Roast Potatoes and a mixed salad. Alternatively, leave until cold and serve with new potatoes and salad.

Poached Chicken with Lemon Sauce

SERVES 4

☀ LOW SATURATED FAT ☀ LOW CHOLESTEROL ☀ SOME FIBRE

4 skinless chicken breasts

*300 ml/½ pt/1¼ cups chicken stock, made with
1 stock cube*

Finely grated rind and juice of 1 small lemon

30 ml/2 tbsp clear honey

1 bay leaf

Freshly ground black pepper

15 ml/1 tbsp cornflour (cornstarch)

15 ml/1 tbsp cold water

30 ml/2 tbsp low-fat fromage frais

30 ml/2 tbsp chopped parsley

Almond Wild Rice (see page 130) and spinach, to serve

1 Put the chicken breasts in a flameproof casserole (Dutch oven). Add the stock, lemon rind and juice, honey, bay leaf and lots of pepper.

2 Bring to the boil, reduce the heat, cover and cook very gently for 15 minutes.

3 Remove the bay leaf, then carefully lift out the chicken breasts. Blend the cornflour with the water and stir in to the cooking juices. Bring to the boil and cook for 1 minute, stirring. Stir in the fromage frais. Return the chicken to the sauce and heat through.

4 Sprinkle the parsley over and serve with Almond Wild Rice and spinach.

Quick Italian Chicken

★ LOW SATURATED FAT ★ LOW CHOLESTEROL ★ NO FIBRE

4 skinless chicken breasts

295 g/10½ oz/1 medium can of half-fat condensed cream of tomato soup

2.5 ml/½ tsp dried basil

Freshly ground black pepper

Broccoli and Sesame Seed Noodles (see page 131), to serve

1 Put the chicken breasts in a non-stick frying pan (skillet).

2 Spoon over the soup. Half-fill the can with water, and pour over. Add the basil and lots of pepper.

3 Bring to the boil, reduce the heat, cover and cook gently for 20 minutes, stirring gently occasionally, until the chicken is cooked through and is bathed in a rich tomato sauce.

4 Serve the chicken with Broccoli and Sesame Seed Noodles.

Chicken Biryani

★ LOW SATURATED FAT ★ LOW CHOLESTEROL ★ HIGH FIBRE

1 quantity of Yellow Rice with Bay (see page 129)

1 onion, sliced

10 ml/2 tsp sunflower oil

225 g/8 oz chicken stir-fry meat

7.5 ml/1½ tsp turmeric

1 garlic clove, crushed

2.5 ml/½ tsp ground ginger

2.5 ml/½ tsp ground cumin

2.5 ml/½ tsp ground coriander (cilantro)

150 ml/¼ pt/⅔ cup low-fat plain yoghurt

A pinch of salt

Freshly ground black pepper

30 ml/2 tbsp currants

30 ml/2 tbsp flaked (slivered) almonds

Green Pepper and Onion Salad (see page 139), to serve

1 Prepare the Yellow Rice with Bay.

2 While it's cooking, fry (sauté) the onion in the oil for 3 minutes. Add the chicken and fry for 3 minutes, stirring.

3 Add the turmeric and all the remaining ingredients, except the currants and almonds. Bring to the boil, then reduce the heat and simmer for about 20 minutes, stirring occasionally, until almost dry (the mixture will curdle at first).

4 Dry-fry the currants and almonds in a frying pan (skillet) until the nuts are golden, stirring all the time.

5 Rinse the Yellow Rice with Bay with boiling water to make a fluffy pilau (see page 129).

6 Serve the chicken on a bed of the rice with the currants and almonds sprinkled over and a Green Pepper and Onion Salad.

Pot Roast Paprika Chicken with Rice

<hr>

SERVES 6

<hr>

★ LOW SATURATED FAT ★ LOW CHOLESTEROL ★ HIGH FIBRE

<hr>

1.5 kg/3 lb oven-ready chicken

15 ml/1 tbsp olive oil

1 onion, finely chopped

1 green (bell) pepper, finely chopped

1 celery stick, chopped

225 g/8 oz/1 cup brown long-grain rice

400 g/14 oz/1 large can of chopped tomatoes

*450 ml/¾ pt/2 cups chicken stock, made with
1 stock cube*

1 bouquet garni sachet

Freshly ground black pepper

15 ml/1 tbsp paprika

200 g/7 oz/1 small can of naturally sweet sweetcorn (corn)

<hr>

1 Remove all the skin from the chicken. Pull off any excess fat just inside the rim of the body cavity.

2 Heat the oil in a large flameproof casserole (Dutch oven) and fry (sauté) the onion, pepper and celery for 2 minutes.

3 Add the rice and stir for 1 minute.

4 Add the tomatoes, stock and bouquet garni and season well with pepper. Top with the chicken and dust the flesh with the paprika.

5 Bring to the boil, cover and place in a preheated oven at 190°C/375°F/gas mark 5. Cook for 1¼ hours. Discard the bouquet garni and stir in the sweetcorn. Re-cover and cook in the oven for a further 15 minutes.

6 Carve the chicken and serve hot with the rice.

Baked Chicken with Orange and Walnuts

SERVES 4

★ LOW SATURATED FAT ★ LOW CHOLESTEROL ★ SOME FIBRE

1 orange

4 skinless chicken breasts

50 g/2 oz/½ cup walnut halves, finely chopped

45 ml/3 tbsp sherry

15 ml/1 tbsp reduced-salt soy sauce

A pinch of chilli powder

A pinch of ground cinnamon

30 ml/2 tbsp clear honey

10 ml/2 tsp cornflour (cornstarch)

15 ml/1 tbsp water

30 ml/2 tbsp chopped parsley, to garnish

New potatoes, boiled in their skins, and Citrus Chinese Leaf Salad (see page 136), to serve

1 Thinly pare the rind from half the orange. Cut into thin strips and boil in water for 1 minute. Drain and reserve. Finely grate the remaining rind and squeeze the juice.

2 Make several slits in each chicken breast and lay in a flameproof casserole (Dutch oven).

3 Mix the chopped nuts with all the remaining ingredients, except the cornflour and water, and spoon over the chicken. Chill for 1 hour to marinate.

4 Bake in a preheated oven at 200°C/400°F/gas mark 6 for 35 minutes until cooked through.

5 Carefully lift the chicken out of the pan and transfer to warm serving plates. Blend the cornflour with the water and stir into the juice. Bring to the boil and cook for 1 minute, stirring.

6 Cut the chicken into slices and fan out on the plates. Spoon the sauce over. Garnish with the reserved orange rind and chopped parsley. Serve with new potatoes in their skins and a Citrus Chinese Leaf Salad.

Chicken Gumbo

SERVES 4

★ LOW SATURATED FAT ★ LOW CHOLESTEROL ★ SOME FIBRE

15 ml/1 tbsp olive oil

450 g/1 lb skinless chicken meat, cut into dice

12 button (pearl) onions, peeled but left whole

*1 rasher (slice) of extra-lean back bacon,
cut into small dice*

5 ml/1 tsp turmeric

5 ml/1 tsp ground coriander (cilantro)

2.5 ml/½ tsp chilli powder

225 g/8 oz okra (ladies' fingers), trimmed

1 red (bell) pepper, sliced

1 green pepper, sliced

225 g/8 oz/1 small can of chopped tomatoes

15 ml/1 tbsp tomato purée (paste)

1 large bay leaf

2.5 ml/½ tsp dried oregano

*600 ml/1 pt/2¼ cups chicken stock, made with
2 stock cubes*

Freshly ground black pepper

15 ml/1 tbsp chopped parsley

Perfect Brown Rice (see page 130), to serve

1 Heat the oil in a large flameproof casserole (Dutch oven). Add the chicken and brown for 3 minutes, stirring.

2 Add the onions, bacon and spices and cook, stirring, for a further 1 minute.

3 Add all the remaining ingredients except the parsley. Bring to the boil, reduce the heat, cover and simmer very gently for 1 hour.

4 Remove the bay leaf. Sprinkle with chopped parsley and serve spooned over the Perfect Brown Rice in large soup bowls.

French-style Peasant Chicken

★ LOW SATURATED FAT ★ LOW CHOLESTEROL ★ SOME FIBRE

If you can't get chanterelles, use button or chestnut mushrooms instead.

450 g/1 lb potatoes, scrubbed and cut into even-sized pieces

15 ml/1 tbsp olive oil

4 chicken portions, skin removed

100g/4 oz chanterelle mushrooms

A pinch of salt

Freshly ground black pepper

150 ml/¼ pt/⅔ cup chicken stock, made with ½ stock cube

1 large garlic clove, finely chopped

30 ml/2 tbsp chopped parsley

Flat Bean Salad (see page 138), to serve

1 Wrap the prepared potatoes in a clean tea towel (dishcloth) to dry while preparing the chicken.

2 Heat the oil in a large non-stick frying pan (skillet) and brown the chicken on all sides.

3 Remove from the pan. Add the potatoes and toss in the pan for about 5 minutes until browning.

4 Add the chanterelles and toss gently. Return the chicken to the pan and sprinkle with a very little salt and lots of pepper. Add 60 ml/4 tbsp of the stock. Cover the pan tightly and turn the heat down low.

5 Cook gently for 45 minutes until everything is tender. Sprinkle the garlic and parsley over and re-cover for a further 5 minutes' cooking time.

6 Carefully lift the chicken, potatoes and chanterelles out of the pan on to warm serving plates and keep warm.

7 Add the remaining stock, boil rapidly for 1 minute to reduce slightly, then spoon over the chicken. Serve straight away with a Flat Bean Salad.

Chicken, Spinach and Pecan Pies

SERVES 4

★ LOW SATURATED FAT ★ LOW CHOLESTEROL ★ SOME FIBRE

2 chicken breasts, cut into small pieces

225 g/8 oz frozen leaf spinach, thawed

100 g/4 oz/½ cup low-fat cottage cheese

25 g/1 oz/¼ cup pecan nuts, chopped

A good pinch of grated nutmeg

Freshly ground black pepper

A pinch of salt

4 large sheets of filo pastry (paste)

10 ml/2 tsp olive oil

Courgettes à la Provençale (see page 134), to serve

1 Put the chicken in a bowl. Squeeze out all excess moisture from the spinach, chop, then add to the chicken with the cheese, nuts, nutmeg, a good grinding of pepper and just a pinch of salt. Mix thoroughly.

2 Lay a sheet of filo pastry on the work surface and brush very lightly with a little of the oil. Fold the pastry in half to form a square. Brush with a little more oil and fold in half again. Add a quarter of the chicken mixture, then fold the pastry over the filling to form a neat parcel.

3 Transfer to a non-stick baking (cookie) sheet and repeat with the remaining ingredients. Brush each parcel with any remaining oil.

4 Bake in a preheated oven at 190°C/375°F/gas mark 5 for 30 minutes until golden and cooked through. Serve with Courgettes à la Provençale.

Barbecued Turkey Steaks

SERVES 4

★ LOW SATURATED FAT ★ LOW CHOLESTEROL ★ NO FIBRE

10 ml/2 tsp sunflower oil

4 turkey breast steaks

15 ml/1 tbsp lemon juice

15 ml/1 tbsp malt vinegar

30 ml/2 tbsp tomato purée (paste)

15 ml/1 tbsp Worcestershire sauce

30 ml/2 tbsp clear honey

Pan-scalloped Potatoes (see page 126) and French (green) beans, to serve

1 Heat the oil in a large non-stick frying pan (skillet). Add the turkey steaks and brown for 1 minute on each side.

2 Mix the remaining ingredients together and spoon over. Cook for about 8 minutes, turning occasionally, over a gentle heat, until the steaks are cooked through and stickily glazed in the sauce.

3 Serve with Pan-scalloped Potatoes and French beans.

Simple Turkey Satay

SERVES 4

★ LOW SATURATED FAT ★ LOW CHOLESTEROL ★ SOME FIBRE

1 shallot, finely chopped

1 large garlic clove, crushed

10 ml/2 tsp sunflower oil

30 ml/2 tbsp smooth wholenut peanut butter

10 ml/2 tsp lime juice

15 ml/1 tbsp clear honey

15 ml/1 tbsp reduced-salt soy sauce

1.5 ml/¼ tsp chilli powder

120 ml/4 fl oz/½ cup skimmed milk

450 g/1 lb thick turkey breast steaks, diced

*175 g/6 oz/¾ cup Thai fragrant rice and Warm
Courgette and Carrot Salad (see page 140),
to serve*

1 Fry (sauté) the shallot and garlic in the oil for 2 minutes, stirring.

2 Stir in all the remaining ingredients except the milk and turkey. Bring to the boil, stirring.

3 Blend in 90 ml/6 tbsp of the milk, reduce the heat and simmer for 2 minutes.

4 Thread the turkey on to soaked wooden skewers. Brush with a little of the sauce.

5 Grill (broil) for about 8 minutes, turning occasionally, until tender and cooked through.

6 Meanwhile, prepare and cook the rice according to the packet directions. Drain.

7 Reheat the remaining sauce with the remaining milk. Lay the kebabs on a bed of the Thai fragrant rice, spoon the remaining sauce over and serve with a Warm Courgette and Carrot Salad.

Kentucky Baked Turkey

SERVES 4

✱ LOW SATURATED FAT ✱ LOW CHOLESTEROL ✱ LOW FIBRE

4 turkey breast steaks

5 ml/1 tsp coarsely ground black pepper

5 ml/1 tsp paprika

5 ml/1 tsp onion powder

1.5 ml/¼ tsp chilli powder

10 ml/2 tsp sunflower oil

4 small bananas

Jacket-baked Potatoes with Yoghurt and Chives (see page 125) and mixed peas and sweetcorn (corn), to serve

1 Beat the turkey steaks briefly to flatten slightly and tenderise.

2 Mix the pepper, paprika and the onion and chilli powders together.

3 Brush the turkey with a little of the oil. Dust with the pepper mixture on each side.

4 Brush a non-stick roasting tin (pan) with some of the remaining oil and lay the turkey in it.

5 Peel and halve the bananas lengthways. Place flat sides down in a small roasting tin, which has been brushed with a little of the remaining oil. Brush with the last of the oil.

6 Bake near the top of a preheated oven at 200°C/ 400°F/gas mark 6 for 20 minutes or until the turkey is tender and cooked through and the bananas have softened slightly.

7 Serve the turkey and bananas with Jacket-baked Potatoes with Yoghurt and Chives and peas with sweetcorn.

Minted Lamb and Vegetable Parcels

SERVES 4

★ LOW SATURATED FAT ★ LOW CHOLESTEROL ★ SOME FIBRE

10 ml/2 tsp sunflower oil

275 g/10 oz lamb fillet, cut into 16 slices

5 ml/1 tsp dried mint

16 small new potatoes, scrubbed

2 small leeks, sliced

4 carrots, sliced

A pinch of salt

Freshly ground black pepper

¼ chicken or beef stock cube

90 ml/6 tbsp boiling water

1 Prepare four pieces of foil about 37.5 cm/15 in square and brush with the oil.

2 Lay four slices of lamb fillet in the centre of each and sprinkle them with a little of the mint. Arrange the vegetables around the meat and sprinkle with salt and pepper.

3 Dissolve the stock cube in the boiling water and pour over the ingredients.

4 Draw the opposite sides of the foil up over the ingredients and fold over to seal. Roll in the edges tightly to seal completely.

5 Transfer to a baking (cookie) sheet and bake in a preheated oven at 190°C/375°F/gas mark 5 for 1 hour. Transfer the parcels to warm plates and open up at the table.

Turkey Stir-fry

SERVES 4

★ LOW SATURATED FAT ★ LOW CHOLESTEROL ★ FAIRLY HIGH FIBRE

15 ml/1 tbsp sunflower oil

175 g/6 oz turkey stir-fry meat

1 onion, thinly sliced

1 large carrot, cut into matchsticks

1 red (bell) pepper, cut into thin strips

1 courgette (zucchini), cut into matchsticks

100 g/4 oz green cabbage, thinly shredded

50 g/2 oz frozen peas

100 g/4 oz/2 cups beansprouts

15 ml/1 tbsp reduced-salt soy sauce

1.5 ml/¼ tsp ground ginger

10 ml/2 tsp clear honey

30 ml/2 tbsp sherry

Freshly ground black pepper

175 g/6 oz wholewheat Chinese egg noodles

1 Heat the oil in a wok or large frying pan (skillet). Add the turkey and stir-fry for 4 minutes. Add the onion and carrot and stir-fry for 2 minutes.

2 Add the remaining vegetables and stir-fry for 3 minutes. Add the flavourings and toss for 2–3 minutes or until the vegetables are cooked to your liking.

3 Meanwhile, cook the noodles according to the packet directions. Drain. Spoon into bowls and top with the Turkey Stir-fry.

Lamb Leg Steaks with Caper Sauce

SERVES 4

★ LOW SATURATED FAT ★ LOW CHOLESTEROL ★ LOW FIBRE

4 lamb leg steaks, trimmed of all fat

Freshly ground black pepper

2.5 ml/½ tsp dried oregano

1 onion, cut into rings

30 ml/2 tbsp cornflour (cornstarch)

100 ml/3½ fl oz/6½ tbsp skimmed milk

*150 ml/¼ pt/⅔ cup lamb or chicken stock,
made with ½ stock cube*

15 ml/1 tbsp chopped parsley

15 ml/1 tbsp capers, chopped

5 ml/1 tsp vinegar from the jar of capers

Sprigs of parsley, to garnish

*Plain boiled potatoes and West Country Carrots
(see page 133), to serve*

1 Place the meat in a non-stick roasting tin (pan). Add a good grinding of pepper and the oregano and top with the onion rings.

2 Cook in the top of a preheated oven at 220°C/425°F/ gas mark 7 for 30 minutes until cooked through.

3 Meanwhile, blend the cornflour in a saucepan with a little of the milk. Stir in the remainder and add the stock. Bring to the boil and cook for 2 minutes, stirring all the time.

4 Stir in the parsley and capers and season to taste with the vinegar and pepper.

5 Transfer the meat to warm plates and spoon any juices over. Garnish with parsley sprigs and serve with the sauce, plain boiled potatoes in their skins and West Country Carrots.

Farmer's Beans

★ LOW SATURATED FAT ★ LOW CHOLESTEROL ★ HIGH FIBRE

*225 g/8 oz/2 cups dried haricot (navy) beans,
soaked in cold water overnight*

450 ml/¾ pt/2 cups water

1 chicken stock cube

10 ml/2 tsp sunflower oil

225 g/8 oz lean shoulder pork, cut into cubes

2 onions, thinly sliced

1 carrot, diced

1 turnip, diced

3 tomatoes, skinned and chopped

15 ml/1 tbsp black treacle (molasses)

2.5 ml/½ tsp dried thyme

Freshly ground black pepper

A pinch of salt

15 ml/1 tbsp chopped parsley, to garnish

1 Drain the beans and place in a large flameproof casserole (Dutch oven). Cover with the water. Bring to the boil and boil rapidly for 10 minutes. Stir in the stock cube.

2 Meanwhile, heat the oil in a non-stick frying pan (skillet). Fry (sauté) the meat and onions, stirring, for 3 minutes. Remove from the pan with a draining spoon.

3 Add the meat, onions and all the remaining ingredients to the beans and bring back to the boil.

4 Cover and place in a preheated oven at 150°C/300°F/gas mark 2 for 4 hours or until the beans are really tender and are bathed in a rich sauce.

5 Sprinkle with parsley and serve hot.

Pork Medallions with Juniper and Port

SERVES 4

☆ LOW SATURATED FAT ☆ LOW CHOLESTEROL ☆ VERY LOW FIBRE

Finely grated rind and juice of ½ lemon

12 juniper berries, crushed

5 ml/1 tsp coarsely ground black peppercorns

275–350 g/10–12 oz pork fillet, cut into 12 slices

15 ml/1 tbsp sunflower oil

1 shallot, finely chopped

10 ml/2 tsp chopped sage

100 ml/3½ fl oz/6½ tbsp port

75 ml/5 tbsp water

½ chicken stock cube

Small sprigs of sage, to garnish

Savoury Potato Cake (see page 124) and broccoli, to serve

1 Mix the lemon rind and juice with the juniper berries and ground peppercorns.

2 Put the pork slices in a plastic bag and beat with a rolling pin or meat mallet to flatten slightly. Coat with the juniper mixture.

3 Heat the oil in a large non-stick frying pan (skillet), and fry (sauté) the pork for 2–3 minutes on each side until cooked through. Transfer to a warm serving dish.

4 Add the shallot and sage to the pan and fry for 1 minute. Add the port, water and stock cube and cook, stirring, until slightly thickened. Spoon over the pork and garnish with small sprigs of sage. Serve with Savoury Potato Cake and broccoli.

Luxury Giant Spring Rolls

SERVES 4

★ LOW SATURATED FAT ★ LOW CHOLESTEROL ★ SOME FIBRE

175 g/6 oz fillet steak, cut into very thin strips

15 ml/1 tbsp cornflour (cornstarch)

20 ml/4 tsp sesame or sunflower oil

1 garlic clove, crushed

4 spring onions (scallions), chopped

4 mushrooms, thinly sliced

100 g/4 oz/2 cups beansprouts

1 carrot, coarsely grated

25 g/1 oz frozen peas

30 ml/2 tbsp reduced-salt soy sauce

1.5 ml/¼ tsp ground ginger

4 sheets of filo pastry (paste)

Citrus Chinese Leaf Salad (see page 136), to serve

1 Mix the beef with the cornflour.

2 Heat half the oil in a large non-stick frying pan (skillet) or wok and stir-fry the meat for 1 minute. Add all the remaining ingredients except the pastry sheets and cook for 3 minutes, stirring. Leave to cool.

3 Lay the pastry sheets on the work surface and fold in half. Divide the mixture into four portions. Place one portion in the centre of one edge of each pastry sheet.

4 Fold in the sides, then roll up.

5 Brush a non-stick baking (cookie) sheet with a little of the remaining oil. Lay the rolls on the sheet and brush with the remaining oil.

6 Bake the rolls on the shelf above the centre, in a preheated oven at 190°C/375°F/gas mark 5 for 20 minutes until golden brown.

7 Serve hot with a Citrus Chinese Leaf Salad.

Grilled Steaks with Mushroom Purée

SERVES 4

★ LOW SATURATED FAT ★ LOW CHOLESTEROL ★ VERY LOW FIBRE

350 g/12 oz button mushrooms, chopped

30 ml/2 tbsp snipped chives

120 ml/4 fl oz/½ cup water

A pinch of salt

Freshly ground black pepper

100 g/4 oz/½ cup low-fat fromage frais

A little skimmed milk

4 small fillet steaks, trimmed of any sinews

5 ml/1 tsp sunflower oil

A few snipped chives, to garnish

*Pan-scalloped Potatoes (see page 126) and
mangetout (snow peas), to serve*

1 Put the mushrooms, chives and water in a pan with the salt and lots of pepper. Bring to the boil, cover, reduce the heat and simmer for 5 minutes until really soft.

2 Purée in a blender or food processor with the fromage frais. Return to the pan. Thin with a little milk, if necessary, then reheat.

3 Meanwhile, put the steaks on a grill (broiler) rack. Brush with the oil and add a good grinding of pepper. Grill (broil) until browned on both sides and cooked to your liking (5–10 minutes).

4 Spoon the purée on to plates, top with a steak and sprinkle with chives. Serve with Pan-scalloped Potatoes and mangetout.

FISH AND VEGETABLE MAIN MEALS

Fish is highly nutritious and great if you want to lower your cholesterol levels as it contains polyunsaturated fats. Oily fish are particularly beneficial. Dried peas, beans and lentils are also very healthy as they are not only a good source of vegetable protein but also high in fibre.

Crab and Spinach Oatmeal Tart

<hr/>

SERVES 6

☀ LOW SATURATED FAT ☀ LOW CHOLESTEROL ☀ HIGH FIBRE

100 g/4 oz/1 cup rolled oats

50 g/2 oz/½ cup wholemeal flour

A pinch of salt

5 ml/1 tsp baking powder

85 g/3½ oz/scant ½ cup sunflower or olive oil spread

Cold water, to mix

Filling:

1 small onion, finely chopped

225 g/8 oz frozen leaf spinach, thawed

170 g/6 oz/1 small can of crabmeat, drained

Finely grated rind of 1 small lemon

40 g/1½ oz/⅓ cup Parmesan cheese, grated

Freshly ground black pepper

1 whole egg

2 egg whites

150 ml/¼ pt/⅔ cup skimmed milk

Tomato and Spring Onion Salad (see page 141), to serve

1 Mix the oats, flour, salt and baking powder together.

2 Add all but 15 g/½ oz/1 tbsp of the spread and rub in with your fingertips. Mix with enough cold water to form a firm dough. Wrap and chill for 30 minutes.

3 Knead gently on a lightly floured surface. Roll out and use to line a 23 cm/9 in flan dish (pie pan).

4 Prick the base with a fork. Line with crumpled foil and bake in a preheated oven at 220°C/425°F/gas mark 7 for 10 minutes. Remove the foil and bake for a further 5 minutes to dry out.

5 Meanwhile, melt the remaining spread in a saucepan. Add the onion and fry (sauté) for 3 minutes, stirring.

6 Squeeze the spinach to remove excess moisture and add to the onion. Cook, stirring, for 3 minutes. Chop up, using scissors.

7 Turn into the flan case (pie shell) and spread out. Top with the crab, sprinkle with the lemon rind, then the cheese and a good grinding of pepper.

8 Whisk the egg, egg whites and milk together and pour into the flan. Bake in the oven at 190°C/375°F/gas mark 5 for 35 minutes until set and golden. Serve warm with a Tomato and Spring Onion Salad.

Baked Cod with Olives and Potatoes

SERVES 4

★ VERY LOW SATURATED FAT ★ LOW CHOLESTEROL ★ SOME FIBRE

4 potatoes, scrubbed and cut into eighths

30 ml/2 tbsp olive oil

4 cod fillets, about 175 g/6 oz each, skinned

10 ml/2 tsp chopped oregano

10 ml/2 tsp chopped parsley

Finely grated rind and juice of ½ lemon

Freshly ground black pepper

1 red onion, chopped

2 ripe beefsteak tomatoes, chopped

1 garlic clove, crushed

16 stoned (pitted) green olives, halved

Dressed Green Salad (see page 137), to serve

1 Boil the potatoes in lightly salted water for 4 minutes until almost tender. Drain.

2 Pour half the oil in a roasting tin (pan), add the potatoes, toss gently and place on the top shelf of an oven preheated to 200°C/400°F/gas mark 6. Cook for 10 minutes.

3 Lay the fish in a separate baking dish, in a single layer. Sprinkle with the herbs, lemon and pepper. Cover with foil and place on the shelf just below the middle of the oven, under the potatoes.

4 Cook for about 30 minutes until the potatoes are turning golden and the fish is tender.

5 Meanwhile, heat the remaining oil in a small pan. Add the onion and fry (sauté), stirring, for 3 minutes. Add the tomatoes, garlic, olives and a good grinding of pepper and simmer, stirring occasionally, for about 5 minutes or until pulpy.

6 When the potatoes and fish are cooked, pour off any juices from the fish into the tomato mixture. Arrange the fish and potatoes on warm serving plates and spoon the tomato sauce over the fish. Serve straight away with a Dressed Green Salad.

Plaice with Grapes

SERVES 4

★ VERY LOW SATURATED FAT ★ LOW CHOLESTEROL ★ LOW FIBRE

4 plaice fillets, cut in half lengthways

*150 ml/¼ pt/⅔ cup chicken stock, made with
½ stock cube*

150 ml/¼ pt/⅔ cup dry white wine

1 small bay leaf

1 small piece of cinnamon stick

150 ml/¼ pt/⅔ cup buttermilk or low-fat crème fraîche

50 g/2 oz seedless green grapes, halved

30 ml/2 tbsp chopped parsley

A pinch of salt

White pepper

*Fluffy Mashed Potatoes (see page 127) and Warm
Courgette and Carrot Salad (see page 140), to serve*

1 Remove any dark skin from the fillets (don't worry if it is white). Roll up, skin-sides in, and place in a single layer in a large, shallow, flameproof dish.

2 Pour over the stock and wine and add the bay leaf and cinnamon. Cover with foil and bake in a preheated oven at 190°C/375°F/gas mark 5 for 15–20 minutes until the fish is cooked through. Carefully lift out the plaice rolls and keep warm.

3 Boil the cooking liquid on top of the stove until it has reduced by half. Discard the bay leaf and cinnamon.

4 Add the buttermilk or crème fraîche, grapes and parsley, season to taste and heat through.

5 Carefully transfer the fish to warm serving plates and spoon the sauce over. Serve hot with Fluffy Mashed Potatoes and a Warm Courgette and Carrot Salad.

Tandoori Fish with Red Rice

SERVES 4

★ VERY LOW SATURATED FAT ★ LOW CHOLESTEROL ★ HIGH FIBRE

450 g/1 lb cod fillet, skinned

150 ml/¼ pt/⅔ cup low-fat plain yoghurt

15 ml/1 tbsp lemon juice

5 ml/1 tsp ground coriander (cilantro)

5 ml/1 tsp ground cumin

2.5 ml/½ tsp turmeric

A pinch of salt

Freshly ground black pepper

175 g/6 oz/¾ cup brown long-grain rice

400 g/14 oz/1 large can of chopped tomatoes

300 ml/½ pt/1¼ cups water

1 vegetable stock cube, crumbled

6 green cardamom pods, split (optional)

2 spring onions (scallions), chopped, to garnish

1 Cut the fish into four equal pieces. Place in a shallow dish in a single layer.

2 Mix the yoghurt with the lemon, spices, salt and pepper. Spoon over the fish and turn gently to coat completely.

3 Cover and leave in a cool place to marinate for 1 hour.

4 Remove the cover and bake in a preheated oven at 180°C/350°F/gas mark 4 for 20 minutes, basting occasionally.

5 Meanwhile, wash the rice and place in a pan with the remaining ingredients. Bring to the boil, reduce the heat and simmer for 35 minutes, adding a little extra water, if necessary, until the rice is tender but nutty and has absorbed all the liquid.

6 Pile the rice on warm plates, top with the fish and garnish with chopped spring onion.

Family Fish Pie

★ VERY LOW SATURATED FAT ★ LOW CHOLESTEROL ★ SOME FIBRE

750 g/1½ lb potatoes, peeled and cut into even-sized pieces

15 g/½ oz/1 tbsp sunflower or olive oil spread

450 g/¾ pt/2 cups skimmed milk

450 g/1 lb white fish fillet, skinned

175 g/6 oz frozen mixed vegetables

1 bouquet garni sachet

A pinch of salt

Freshly ground black pepper

45 ml/3 tbsp plain (all-purpose) flour

30 ml/2 tbsp chopped parsley

A little paprika

1 Cook the potatoes in boiling, lightly salted water until tender. Drain and mash with the low-fat spread and 30 ml/2 tbsp of the milk.

2 Meanwhile, put the fish in a flameproof casserole (Dutch oven) with the remaining milk and the mixed vegetables. Add the bouquet garni, salt and some pepper. Bring to the boil, reduce the heat, cover and simmer for 7–8 minutes until just tender.

3 Blend the flour with a little water in a cup. Stir into the fish mixture. Bring to the boil and simmer for 2 minutes, stirring until thickened. Add the parsley, taste and re-season, if necessary.

4 Pile the mashed potato on top and sprinkle with paprika. Place under a hot grill (broiler) until golden and bubbling. Serve straight away.

Speciality Trout with Almonds

★ VERY LOW SATURATED FAT ★ LOW CHOLESTEROL ★ SOME FIBRE

15 g/½ oz/1 tbsp sunflower or olive oil spread

*4 rainbow trout, cleaned and heads removed,
if preferred*

120 ml/4 fl oz/½ cup medium cider

30 ml/2 tbsp toasted flaked (slivered) almonds

15 ml/1 tbsp chopped parsley

15 ml/1 tbsp snipped chives

Freshly ground black pepper

*New potatoes, boiled in their skins, and
French (green) beans, to serve*

1 Melt the spread in a large non-stick frying pan (skillet). Add the trout and fry (sauté) for 5 minutes on each side until cooked through.

2 Lift out of the pan with a fish slice and transfer to warm serving plates. Keep warm.

3 Add the cider to the juices in the pan and boil, stirring, until reduced by half. Add the nuts and herbs and a good grinding of pepper. Stir well, then spoon over the trout.

4 Serve straight away with new potatoes in their skins and French beans.

Soused Mackerel

SERVES 4

★ VERY LOW SATURATED FAT ★ LOW CHOLESTEROL ★ VERY LOW FIBRE

4 mackerel, cleaned and heads removed

2 small onions

4 small sprigs of dill (dill weed)

15 ml/1 tbsp pickling spices

1 bay leaf

120 ml/4 fl oz/½ cup malt vinegar

120 ml/4 fl oz/½ cup water

10 ml/2 tsp clear honey

1.5 ml/¼ tsp salt

New potatoes, boiled in their skins, and Blushing Leaf Salad (see page 142), to serve

1 Lay the fish flat on a board, skin-sides up. Run your thumb up and down each backbone firmly to loosen it. Turn the fish over and carefully lift off the backbones, removing any loose bones as well.

2 Finely chop one of the onions. Scatter over the fish and lay a sprig of dill on each. Roll up. Place in an ovenproof dish.

3 Slice the remaining onion and separate into rings. Scatter over with the pickling spices and the bay leaf, broken in half.

4 Mix the vinegar and water, honey and salt together and pour over. Cover with foil and bake in a preheated oven at 160°C/325°F/gas mark 3 for about 1 hour or until the fish is cooked through. Remove from the oven and leave to cool in the liquid.

5 Chill. Remove from the marinade with a draining spoon and serve cold with new potatoes in their skins and a Blushing Leaf Salad.

⤳

Fast Mixed-bean Chilli

SERVES 4

★ VERY LOW SATURATED FAT ★ NO CHOLESTEROL ★ HIGH FIBRE

1 onion, finely chopped

1 red (bell) pepper, finely chopped

15 g/½ oz/1 tbsp sunflower or olive oil spread

5 ml/1 tsp ground cumin

5 ml/1 tsp dried oregano

2.5 ml/½ tsp hot chilli powder (or to taste)

400 g/14 oz/1 large can of chopped tomatoes

2 × 425 g/15 oz/large cans of mixed pulses, drained

Oat Tortillas (see page 161), shredded lettuce and chopped cucumber, to serve

1 Fry (sauté) the onion and red pepper in the spread, stirring, for 3 minutes.

2 Add the cumin, oregano and chilli powder and stir for 1 minute.

3 Add the chopped tomatoes and drained pulses. Cook, stirring, for 10 minutes until they are bathed in a rich sauce.

4 Spoon on to Oat Tortillas, top with some shredded lettuce and chopped cucumber, roll up and serve. Eat with your fingers.

Smoked Haddock-stuffed Pancakes

SERVES 4

★ VERY LOW SATURATED FAT ★ LOW CHOLESTEROL ★ HIGH FIBRE

1 quantity of Oat Bran and Wholemeal Pancakes
(see page 162)

Filling:

225 g/8 oz undyed smoked haddock, skinned

100 g/4 oz button mushrooms, sliced

350 ml/12 fl oz/1½ cups skimmed milk

45 ml/3 tbsp plain (all-purpose) flour

5 ml/1 tsp lemon juice

30 ml/2 tbsp chopped parsley

Freshly ground black pepper

Lemon wedges and sprigs of parsley, to garnish

Mangetout (snow peas) and baby carrots, to serve

1 Prepare and cook the pancakes, then keep them warm over a pan of hot water.

2 Make the filling. Poach the fish and mushrooms in 300 ml/½ pt/1¼ cups of the milk for 6 minutes or until the fish flakes easily with a fork. Lift the fish out of the milk and reserve.

3 Blend the flour with the remaining milk. Stir into the fish milk, bring to the boil and cook for 2 minutes, stirring until thickened.

4 Add the lemon juice, parsley and pepper to taste. Flake the fish and fold in gently. Heat through, stirring lightly, until piping hot.

5 Divide the mixture among the pancakes, roll up and arrange on warm plates. Garnish with lemon wedges and sprigs of parsley and serve straight away with mangetout and baby carrots.

⤳

Spaghetti with Cherry Tomatoes and Pesto

SERVES 4

★ VERY LOW SATURATED FAT ★ NO CHOLESTEROL ★ HIGH FIBRE

350 g/12 oz wholewheat spaghetti

1 quantity of Simple Pesto (see page 177)

100 g/4 oz cherry tomatoes, halved

50 g/2 oz stoned (pitted) black olives, halved

60 ml/4 tbsp boiling water

15 ml/1 tbsp olive oil

1 Cook the spaghetti according to the packet directions. Drain and return to the pan.

2 Add the Simple Pesto and toss gently.

3 Add the tomatoes, olives and boiling water and continue tossing over a gentle heat for about 3 minutes, until the tomatoes are just softening.

4 Pile on to warm plates and drizzle with the olive oil before serving.

Leek and Corn Stuffed Potatoes

SERVES 4

★ VERY LOW SATURATED FAT ★ LOW CHOLESTEROL ★ HIGH FIBRE

4 large potatoes, scrubbed

2 leeks, thinly sliced

90 ml/6 tbsp skimmed milk

A pinch of salt

Freshly ground black pepper

15 g/½ oz/1 tbsp sunflower or olive oil spread

*200 g/7 oz/1 small can of naturally sweet
sweetcorn (corn), drained*

4 small, ripe tomatoes

50 g/2 oz/½ cup low-fat Cheddar cheese, grated

English Mixed Salad (see page 140), to serve

1 Prick the potatoes all over. Bake in a preheated oven at 180°C/350°F/gas mark 4 for 1½ hours or until soft when squeezed.

2 Meanwhile, put the leeks and milk in a saucepan. Bring to the boil, reduce the heat, cover and cook very gently for 10 minutes until the leeks are soft.

3 Cut a slice off the top of each potato and scoop most of the soft flesh out into a bowl.

4 Add the leeks and their milk, the salt, a good grinding of pepper and the spread and mash thoroughly. Stir in the sweetcorn.

5 Spoon half the potato mixture back into the skins and press down well. Add a ripe tomato to each, then a good grinding of pepper. Spoon over the remaining potato mixture and roughen the top with a fork.

6 Place on a baking (cookie) sheet and sprinkle with the cheese. Top with the potato lids. Return to the oven for 30 minutes until piping hot and golden brown. Serve hot with an English Mixed Salad.

Pappardelle with Roast Mediterranean Vegetables

SERVES 4

★ VERY LOW SATURATED FAT ★ VERY LOW CHOLESTEROL ★ SOME FIBRE

1 aubergine (eggplant), sliced

1 red (bell) pepper, cut into thick strips

1 green pepper, cut into thick strips

1 yellow or orange pepper, cut into thick strips

1 large courgette (zucchini), cut into chunks

1 red onion, cut into eighths

1 garlic clove, crushed

30 ml/2 tbsp olive oil

Freshly ground black pepper

30 ml/2 tbsp pine nuts

250 g/9 oz pappardelle (wide ribbon noodles)

A few thin shavings of Parmesan cheese

1 Plunge all the prepared vegetables in boiling water for 3 minutes. Drain and dry on kitchen paper (paper towels).

2 Arrange in a single layer in a non-stick roasting tin (pan).

3 Mix the garlic and oil together and brush all over. Add a good grinding of pepper.

4 Roast towards the top of a preheated oven at 200°C/400°F/gas mark 6 for 40 minutes until tender and colouring slightly round the edges.

5 Meanwhile, dry-fry the pine nuts in a small frying pan (skillet), tossing until golden brown.

6 Cook the pappardelle according to the packet directions. Drain and pile on to four warm serving plates.

7 Spoon the vegetables over and sprinkle with the pine nuts and Parmesan shavings.

Lentil and Mushroom Madras

SERVES 4

★ VERY LOW SATURATED FAT ★ NO CHOLESTEROL ★ HIGH FIBRE

225 g/8 oz brown lentils

1 large onion, thinly sliced

15 ml/1 tbsp sunflower or olive oil

15 ml/1 tbsp Madras curry powder

175 g/6 oz button mushrooms, halved or quartered

2 large carrots, coarsely grated

*30 ml/2 tbsp mango or curried fruit chutney,
chopped, if necessary*

30 ml/2 tbsp chopped coriander (cilantro)

A pinch of salt

*300 ml/½ pt/1¼ cups vegetable stock,
made with 1 stock cube*

1 bay leaf

5 ml/1 tsp garam masala

*Sliced cucumber and a few sprigs of coriander,
to garnish*

Perfect Brown Rice (see page 130), to serve

1 Soak the lentils in cold water for several hours. Drain and place in a saucepan. Cover with water, bring to the boil and boil for about 45 minutes until really tender. Drain.

2 Fry (sauté) the onion in the oil in a saucepan for 3 minutes. Stir in the curry powder, mushrooms and carrots and continue cooking for 1 minute, stirring.

3 Add all the remaining ingredients except the garam masala, and stir in the cooked lentils.

4 Simmer for about 30 minutes, until the mixture is thick and well flavoured, stirring occasionally.

5 Discard the bay leaf and stir in the garam masala. Taste and re-season, if necessary.

6 Serve garnished with sliced cucumber and sprigs of coriander on a bed of Perfect Brown Rice.

Nut Moussaka

SERVES 4

★ VERY LOW SATURATED FAT ★ VERY LOW CHOLESTEROL ★ HIGH FIBRE

---

2 aubergines (eggplants), sliced

100 g/4 oz/2 cups fresh wholemeal breadcrumbs

1 garlic clove, crushed

90 ml/6 tbsp red wine

60 ml/4 tbsp water

30 ml/2 tbsp olive oil

5 ml/1 tsp dried oregano

30 ml/2 tbsp tomato purée (paste)

200 g/7 oz/1¾ cups chopped mixed nuts

Freshly ground black pepper

30 ml/2 tbsp plain (all-purpose) flour

300 ml/½ pt/1¼ cups skimmed milk

15 g/½ oz/1 tbsp sunflower or olive oil spread

2.5 ml/½ tsp ground cinnamon

A pinch of salt

50 g/2 oz/½ cup low-fat strong Cheddar cheese, grated

Dressed Green Salad (see page 137), to serve

1 Boil the aubergine slices in water for 3 minutes until almost tender. Drain, rinse with cold water and drain again.

2 Meanwhile, mix the next eight ingredients together and season with pepper.

3 Put the flour in a saucepan and gradually stir in the milk until smooth. Add the spread and cinnamon. Bring to the boil and cook for 2 minutes, stirring until thickened. Season with a pinch of salt and some pepper.

4 Layer the aubergine slices and nut mixture in a 1.5 litre/2½ pt/6 cup ovenproof dish.

5 Spoon the sauce over and sprinkle with the cheese. Bake in a preheated oven at 200°C/400°F/gas mark 6 for 35 minutes until the top is golden and bubbling. Serve hot with a Dressed Green Salad.

Spinach and Hazelnut Parcels

SERVES 4

★ VERY LOW SATURATED FAT ★ VERY LOW CHOLESTEROL ★ HIGH FIBRE

450 g/1 lb spinach

1 large red onion, roughly chopped

15 g/½ oz/1 tbsp sunflower or olive oil spread

175 g/6 oz/1½ cups hazelnuts

4 slices of wholemeal bread

1 egg white

5 ml/1 tsp Marmite or Vegemite

90 ml/6 tbsp boiling water

2.5 ml/½ tsp dried mixed herbs

A pinch of salt

Freshly ground black pepper

300 ml/½ pt/1¼ cups passata (sieved tomatoes)

30 ml/2 tbsp chopped parsley

1 garlic clove, crushed

5 ml/1 tsp clear honey

60 ml/4 tbsp low-fat plain yoghurt

Perfect Brown Rice (see page 130), to serve

1 Select 12 of the largest spinach leaves and reserve. Discard the thick central stalks from the remainder. Wash the leaves, shake off the excess water, tear up and place in a saucepan. Cover and cook gently for 5 minutes until tender. Drain off any liquid.

2 Cook the onion gently in the spread for 3 minutes, stirring, until softened. Turn into a food processor with the cooked spinach, nuts and torn-up slices of bread. Run the machine briefly to chop, not too finely.

3 Add the egg white. Dissolve the Marmite or Vegemite in the water. Add to the mixture with the herbs, salt and pepper. Mix gently but thoroughly.

4 Cut off the thick stalks from the reserved spinach leaves. Blanch the leaves briefly in boiling water for 30 seconds. Drain, rinse with cold water and drain again.

5 Open the leaves out on a work surface and divide the nut mixture among them. Fold in the sides, then roll up and lay in an ovenproof dish. Add the remaining water to the dish.

6 Cover with foil or a lid and bake in a preheated oven at 180°C/350°F/gas mark 4 for about 35 minutes until cooked through.

7 Meanwhile, blend the passata with half the parsley, the garlic, honey and a little pepper in the spinach cooking saucepan. Heat through, stirring.

8 Spoon the sauce on to warm serving plates and lay the spinach parcels on top. Spoon a little yoghurt over each parcel, garnish with the remainder of the parsley and serve with Perfect Brown Rice.

Soya Bean Risotto

SERVES 4–6

★ VERY LOW SATURATED FAT ★ VERY LOW CHOLESTEROL ★ HIGH FIBRE

1 onion, chopped

25 g/1 oz/2 tbsp sunflower or olive oil spread

1 carrot, chopped

2 celery sticks, chopped

1 red (bell) pepper, diced

100 g/4 oz frozen peas

75 g/3 oz button mushrooms, sliced

225 g/8 oz/1 cup brown long-grain rice

*600 ml/1pt/2½ cups vegetable stock,
made with 2 stock cubes*

15 ml/1 tbsp reduced-salt soy sauce

15 ml/1 tbsp tomato purée (paste)

5 ml/1 tsp dried mixed herbs

Freshly ground black pepper

*200 g/7 oz/1 small can of naturally sweet
sweetcorn (corn)*

*425 g/15 oz/1 large can of soya beans,
rinsed and drained*

30 ml/2 tbsp pumpkin seeds

1 Fry (sauté) the onion in the spread for 2 minutes in a large non-stick frying pan (skillet).

2 Add the carrot, celery, pepper, peas, mushrooms and rice and cook for 1 minute, stirring.

3 Add the remaining ingredients except the sweetcorn, soya beans and pumpkin seeds. Bring to the boil, reduce the heat, cover and cook gently for about 30 minutes, stirring occasionally, until the rice is tender but nutty and has absorbed the liquid.

4 Add the contents of the can of sweetcorn, the beans and the pumpkin seeds. Cover and cook for 5 minutes. Fork through and serve.

Vitality Fish and Chips

SERVES 4

★ VERY LOW SATURATED FAT ★ LOW CHOLESTEROL ★ SOME FIBRE

4 cod or haddock fillets, about 175 g/6 oz each

75 g/3 oz/1½ cups fresh wholemeal breadcrumbs

5 ml/1 tsp dried mixed herbs

15 ml/1 tbsp dried onion granules

Freshly ground black pepper

1 egg white

15 ml/1 tbsp water

450 g/1 lb frozen chips (French fries), NOT oven chips

Lemon wedges and sprigs of parsley, to garnish

Peas, to serve

1 Remove the skin from the fish fillets and wipe with kitchen paper (paper towels).

2 Mix the breadcrumbs, herbs and onion granules in a shallow dish. Add a good grinding of pepper.

3 Lightly beat the egg white with the water in a dish.

4 Dip the fish in the egg white and then the crumb mix to coat completely.

5 Put the chips in a single layer on a baking (cookie) sheet.

6 Place the chips on the top shelf and the fish just below in a preheated oven at 220°C/425°F/gas mark 7 for 30 minutes until the chips and the fish are cooked and golden. Transfer to warm plates, garnish with lemon wedges and sprigs of parsley and serve with peas.

SIDE DISHES AND SALADS

All these dishes make delicious accompaniments to the main courses in this book. They are also a wonderful way of turning a simple grilled steak, chicken breast or fish fillet into a gourmet meal.

Savoury Potato Cake

SERVES 4

★ VERY LOW SATURATED FAT ★ NO CHOLESTEROL ★ FAIRLY HIGH FIBRE

450 g/1 lb potatoes, scrubbed and grated

1 small onion, grated

A pinch of salt

Freshly ground black pepper

15 ml/1 tbsp sunflower oil

1 Squeeze the grated potato to remove excess moisture. Mix with the grated onion and season with the salt and lots of pepper.

2 Heat half the oil in a medium non-stick frying pan (skillet).

3 Add the potato mixture and press down well. Cover with a lid and cook over a moderate heat for 30 minutes until tender and the base is golden brown.

4 Loosen the potato cake with a spatula. Turn out on to a plate.

5 Heat the remaining oil in the pan, slide the potato cake back in and cook for a further 5–10 minutes over a fairly high heat until browned on the base. Slide out on to a plate and serve cut into wedges.

Jacket-baked Potatoes with Yoghurt and Chives

SERVES 4

★ VERY LOW SATURATED FAT ★ VERY LOW CHOLESTEROL ★ HIGH FIBRE

You can cook these in a high or low oven to suit what else you are cooking. Simply adjust the cooking time accordingly. If your main course is not going to take as long as the potatoes, pop them in the oven before starting to prepare the rest of the meal.

4 fairly large potatoes, scrubbed

5 ml/1 tsp olive oil

90 ml/6 tbsp low-fat plain yoghurt

30 ml/2 tbsp snipped chives

A pinch of salt

Freshly ground black pepper

Paprika for dusting

1 Prick the potatoes all over. Brush with oil.

2 Place on a baking (cookie) sheet and bake in a preheated oven at 180°C/350°F/gas mark 4 for about 1½ hours or until really tender when squeezed. Alternatively, bake in the microwave according to the manufacturer's instructions.

3 Meanwhile, mix the yoghurt with the chives and season with the salt and some pepper. Chill until ready to serve.

4 When the potatoes are cooked, make a cross-cut in the top of each potato and squeeze gently on either side to open up slightly. Transfer to serving plates, spoon the yoghurt and chive mixture over and dust with paprika before serving. Don't forget to eat the skins!

Pan-scalloped Potatoes

SERVES 4

☆ VERY LOW SATURATED FAT ☆ VERY LOW CHOLESTEROL ☆ HIGH FIBRE

450 g/1 lb potatoes, thickly sliced

15 g/½ oz/1 tbsp sunflower or olive oil spread

A pinch of salt

Freshly ground black pepper

30 ml/2 tbsp chopped parsley

150 ml/¼ pt/⅔ cup skimmed milk

1 Boil the potatoes in lightly salted water for 3 minutes. Drain.

2 Grease a flameproof casserole (Dutch oven) with the spread. Lay the potatoes in the casserole, seasoning each layer and sprinkling with parsley.

3 Pour over the milk. Cover with the lid and cook over a very gentle heat for about 40 minutes until cooked through. Serve straight from the pan.

Fluffy Mashed Potatoes

SERVES 4

★ VERY LOW SATURATED FAT ★ ALMOST NO CHOLESTEROL ★ LOW FIBRE

450 g/1 lb potatoes

Salt

15 g/½ oz/1 tbsp sunflower or olive oil spread

A pinch of ground nutmeg

Freshly ground black pepper

30 ml/2 tbsp skimmed milk

1 Peel the potatoes and cut into even-sized pieces.

2 Cook in boiling, lightly salted water until tender. Drain thoroughly.

3 Add the spread, nutmeg, some pepper and the milk. Using an electric beater, beat the mixture thoroughly until smooth and fluffy. Serve straight away.

Seeded Roast Potatoes

SERVES 4

★ VERY LOW SATURATED FAT ★ NO CHOLESTEROL ★ HIGH FIBRE

4 fairly large potatoes, scrubbed and quartered

15 ml/1 tbsp sunflower or olive oil

15 ml/1 tbsp sesame seeds

15 ml/1 tbsp poppy seeds

A pinch of salt

Freshly ground black pepper

1 Put the potatoes in a small roasting tin (pan). Add the oil and toss gently until each piece is coated.

2 Sprinkle with the seeds and a pinch of salt.

3 Bake towards the top of a preheated oven at 200°C/400°F/gas mark 6 for about 1 hour or until golden and cooked through. Sprinkle with pepper and serve hot.

Yellow Rice with Bay Leaves

SERVES 4

★ ALMOST NO SATURATED FAT ★ NO CHOLESTEROL ★ HIGH FIBRE

75 g/3 oz/⅓ cup brown long-grain rice

75 g/3 oz/⅓ cup basmati rice

10 ml/2 tsp turmeric

1 vegetable stock cube, crumbled

1 large bay leaf, torn in half

Freshly ground black pepper

1 yellow (bell) pepper, finely chopped

1 Rinse the brown rice thoroughly, drain well and place in a large non-stick saucepan. Cover with boiling water. Bring back to the boil, cover and cook over a moderate heat for 15 minutes.

2 Meanwhile, rinse the basmati rice and drain well. Add to the brown rice and, again, just cover with boiling water. Stir in the remaining ingredients, cover and cook for a further 10 minutes or until both types of rice are just tender, topping up with a little more boiling water, if necessary.

3 Remove the lid and boil rapidly, if necessary, to remove any excess liquid and serve hot as a moist risotto. Alternatively, to make a pilau, turn the cooked rice into a colander, rinse thoroughly with boiling water, drain and fluff up with a fork. Discard the bay leaf before serving.

Perfect Brown Rice

SERVES 4–6

★ ALMOST NO SATURATED FAT ★ NO CHOLESTEROL ★ HIGH FIBRE

225 g/8 oz/1 cup brown long-grain rice

300 ml/½ pt/1¼ cups water

A pinch of salt

Freshly ground black pepper

Paprika, to garnish

1 Rinse the rice thoroughly and drain well.

2 Put the water in a non-stick saucepan and bring to the boil. Add the rice, stir well, reduce the heat, cover and simmer very gently for 30 minutes.

3 Season well with the salt and lots of pepper and fluff up with a fork. Serve sprinkled with a fine dusting of paprika.

Almond Wild Rice

SERVES 4

★ ALMOST NO SATURATED FAT ★ NO CHOLESTEROL ★ HIGH FIBRE

175 g/6 oz/¾ cup wild rice mix

50 g/2 oz frozen peas

45 ml/3 tbsp flaked (slivered) almonds

30 ml/2 tbsp currants

Freshly ground black pepper

1 Cook the rice according to the packet directions, adding the peas for the last 5 minutes' cooking time. Drain thoroughly.

2 Meanwhile, dry-fry the almonds in a non-stick frying pan (skillet) until golden, stirring all the time to prevent burning. Remove from the pan as soon as they are brown.

3 Add to the rice with the currants and season well with pepper. Toss and serve.

Broccoli and Sesame Seed Noodles

SERVES 4

★ VERY LOW SATURATED FAT ★ NO CHOLESTEROL ★ HIGH FIBRE

225 g/8 oz wholewheat tagliatelle

175 g/6 oz broccoli, cut into tiny florets

45 ml/3 tbsp sesame seeds

15 ml/1 tbsp olive or sesame oil

1 Cook the tagliatelle according to the packet directions, adding the broccoli for the last 4 minutes of cooking time. Drain and return to the saucepan.

2 Meanwhile, dry-fry the sesame seeds in a non-stick frying pan (skillet) until golden.

3 Add to the pasta with the oil, toss and serve.

Tomato Spaghetti

SERVES 4

✱ ALMOST NO SATURATED FAT ✱ NO CHOLESTEROL ✱ HIGH FIBRE

225 g/8 oz wholewheat spaghetti

300 ml/½ pt/1¼ cups passata (sieved tomatoes)

30 ml/2 tbsp chopped basil

Freshly ground black pepper

A few basil leaves, to garnish

1 Cook the spaghetti according to the packet directions. Drain and return to the saucepan.

2 Add the passata, basil and some pepper and toss over a gentle heat until hot through.

3 Serve straight away, garnished with a few extra basil leaves.

West Country Carrots

SERVES 4

★ NO SATURATED FAT ★ NO CHOLESTEROL ★ SOME FIBRE

450 g/1 lb carrots, cut into matchsticks

300 ml/½ pt/1¼ cups medium cider

15 ml/1 tbsp clear honey

A pinch of salt

Freshly ground black pepper

1 Put the carrots in a saucepan with the cider, honey and salt.

2 Bring to the boil, cover, reduce the heat and simmer gently for 20 minutes until the carrots are just tender and the liquid has evaporated, removing the lid for the last 3 minutes of cooking time.

3 Add a good grinding of pepper and serve hot.

Courgettes à la Provençale

SERVES 4

✱   VERY LOW SATURATED FAT   ✱   NO CHOLESTEROL

1 onion, finely chopped

1 garlic clove, crushed

15 ml/1 tbsp sunflower or olive oil

400 g/14 oz/1 large can of chopped tomatoes

4 courgettes (zucchini), sliced

2.5 ml/½ tsp dried mixed herbs

A pinch of salt

Freshly ground black pepper

1 Fry (sauté) the onion and garlic in the oil in a saucepan for 2 minutes, stirring.

2 Add the remaining ingredients. Bring to the boil, reduce the heat and simmer for 15 minutes, stirring occasionally, until the courgettes are just tender and bathed in a rich tomato sauce.

3 Taste and re-season, if necessary.

Caraway Cabbage

SERVES 4

★ ALMOST NO SATURATED FAT ★ NO CHOLESTEROL ★ HIGH FIBRE

*150 ml/¼ pt/⅔ cup chicken or vegetable stock,
made with ½ stock cube*

450 g/1 lb green cabbage, very finely shredded

15 ml/1 tbsp caraway seeds

Freshly ground black pepper

1 Put the stock in a saucepan and bring to the boil.

2 Add the cabbage and stir well.

3 Cover tightly and boil for 5 minutes, shaking the pan occasionally, until the cabbage is still bright green and just tender but has some 'bite'.

4 Season with the caraway seeds and pepper and serve straight away.

Citrus Chinese Leaf Salad

SERVES 4

★ VERY LOW SATURATED FAT ★ NO CHOLESTEROL ★ SOME FIBRE

½ small head of Chinese leaves (stem lettuce)

1 pink grapefruit

2 oranges

15 ml/1 tbsp olive or sunflower oil

A few drops of reduced-salt soy sauce

10 ml/2 tsp lemon juice

Freshly ground black pepper

15 ml/1 tbsp snipped chives, to garnish

1 Cut the Chinese leaves into chunks and place in a shallow dish.

2 Holding the fruit over a bowl to catch the juice, cut off all the skin and pith from the grapefruit and oranges. Cut the grapefruit in segments away from the sides of each membrane. Lay the fruit over the Chinese leaves. Squeeze the membranes over the bowl to catch any remaining juice. Slice the oranges and cut the slices into halves, if liked. Arrange over the leaves.

3 Add the oil, soy sauce and lemon juice to the juices in the bowl and whisk well. Season with pepper.

4 Drizzle over the salad and sprinkle with chives before serving.

Dressed Green Salad

SERVES 4

★ VERY LOW SATURATED FAT ★ NO CHOLESTEROL ★ SOME FIBRE

1 Little Gem lettuce

1 small avocado

Lemon juice

5 cm/2 in piece of cucumber, sliced

1 green (bell) pepper, cut into thin strips

4 spring onions (scallions), cut into short lengths

*A few small sprigs of coriander (cilantro),
torn into pieces*

A few small sprigs of parsley, torn into pieces

1 quantity of Lo-French Dressing (see page 185)

1 Separate the lettuce into leaves, tear into pieces and place in a salad bowl

2 Halve the avocado, remove the stone (pit), peel and slice. Toss gently in lemon juice to prevent browning. Scatter over the lettuce.

3 Scatter the remaining salad ingredients over, then drizzle with the dressing.

4 Toss gently and serve.

Flat Bean Salad

SERVES 4

★ VERY LOW SATURATED FAT ★ NO CHOLESTEROL ★ SOME FIBRE

175 g/6 oz flat green beans

A pinch of salt

1 small red onion, very finely chopped

15 ml/1 tbsp olive oil

10 ml/2 tsp red wine vinegar

Freshly ground black pepper

15 ml/1 tbsp chopped parsley, to garnish

1 Cut the beans into 2.5 cm/1 in lengths.

2 Cook in boiling, lightly salted water for 5 minutes until just tender. Drain, rinse with cold water and drain again.

3 Place in a shallow dish. Sprinkle with the chopped onion.

4 Drizzle the oil and vinegar over and add a good grinding of pepper. Toss gently and chill for at least 30 minutes to allow the flavours to develop. Sprinkle with parsley before serving.

Green Pepper and Onion Salad

SERVES 4

★ VERY LOW SATURATED FAT ★ NO CHOLESTEROL ★ SOME FIBRE

2 large green (bell) peppers, sliced into rings

1 white onion, sliced into rings

1 red onion, sliced into rings

5 ml/1 tsp chopped sage

Freshly ground black pepper

1 quantity of Honey Nut Dressing (see page 184)

1 small sprig of sage, to garnish

1 Plunge the pepper rings into boiling water for 30 seconds. Drain, rinse with cold water and drain again. Place in a salad bowl.

2 Add the onion rings and sprinkle with the sage and lots of pepper.

3 Drizzle the dressing over, toss gently and chill for at least 30 minutes to allow the flavours to develop.

4 Garnish with a small sprig of sage before serving.

English Mixed Salad

SERVES 4

★ VERY LOW SATURATED FAT ★ VERY LOW CHOLESTEROL ★ SOME FIBRE

½ round lettuce

5 cm/2 in piece of cucumber, sliced

2 tomatoes, cut into small wedges

2 spring onions (scallions), chopped

1 small bunch of radishes, trimmed and halved

2 celery sticks, sliced

1 quantity of Gran's Light Dressing (see page 186)

1 Tear the lettuce leaves into bite-sized pieces and place in a salad bowl.

2 Scatter the remaining ingredients over and serve with the dressing handed separately.

Warm Courgette and Carrot Salad

SERVES 4

★ VERY LOW SATURATED FAT ★ NO CHOLESTEROL ★ SOME FIBRE

2 courgettes (zucchini)

2 carrots

30 ml/2 tbsp sunflower oil

30 ml/2 tbsp black mustard seeds

15 ml/1 tbsp lemon juice

5 ml/1 tsp clear honey

1 Coarsely grate the courgettes and carrots into a salad bowl. Mix well.

2 When ready to serve, heat the oil in a frying pan (skillet). Add the seeds and cook until they start to pop.

3 Quickly stir in the lemon juice and honey and drizzle over the vegetables. Toss and serve straight away.

Tomato and Spring Onion Salad

SERVES 4

★ VERY LOW SATURATED FAT ★ VERY LOW CHOLESTEROL ★ SOME FIBRE

2–3 beefsteak tomatoes, halved and sliced

6 spring onions (scallions), finely chopped

15 ml/1 tbsp cider or wine vinegar

Freshly ground black pepper

1 quantity of Light Cheese Dressing (see page 185)

1 Arrange the tomatoes attractively in four small salad bowls.

2 Sprinkle the spring onions over and drizzle with the vinegar. Season with pepper.

3 Just before serving, spoon the Light Cheese Dressing over and serve.

Blushing Leaf Salad

SERVES 4

★ VERY LOW SATURATED FAT ★ VERY LOW CHOLESTEROL ★ SOME FIBRE

1 small head of radicchio

½ lollo rosso lettuce

2 small cooked beetroot (red beets), diced

4 cherry tomatoes, halved

8 radishes, sliced

1 red onion, finely chopped

15 ml/1 tbsp red wine vinegar

Freshly ground black pepper

1 quantity of Rosy Dressing (see page 186), to serve

1 Separate the radicchio and lollo rosso into leaves. Tear into neat pieces and lay on a flat platter.

2 Arrange the remaining ingredients in neat piles on the leaves and sprinkle with the vinegar and pepper.

3 Serve with the dressing handed separately.

DELECTABLE DESSERTS

For many people a meal is not complete without a pud. And just because you are reducing your intake of cholesterol doesn't mean depriving yourself of all your favourite and sinful afters. I have created recipes for everything from Spotted Dick to profiteroles for you to enjoy. But if you don't fancy a full-blown dessert, treat yourself to some exotic fresh fruit, carefully prepared and presented prettily on a plate with a dollop of the lowest-fat crème fraîche, fromage frais or vanilla yoghurt on the side to dip into … heaven!

Spotted Dick

SERVES 4

★ VERY LOW SATURATED FAT ★ VERY LOW CHOLESTEROL ★ HIGH FIBRE

50 g/2 oz/½ cup self-raising (self-rising) wholemeal flour

50 g/2 oz/½ cup self-raising white flour

5 ml/1 tsp baking powder

75 g/3 oz/⅓ cup sunflower or olive oil spread

100 g/4 oz/2 cups fresh wholemeal breadcrumbs

1.5 ml/¼ tsp ground cinnamon

50 g/2 oz/¼ cup caster (superfine) sugar

*150 g/5 oz/scant 1 cup mixed dried fruit
(fruit cake mix) or raisins*

2 egg whites, lightly beaten

100 ml/3½ fl oz/6½ tbsp skimmed milk

A very little sunflower oil for greasing

Low-fat Custard (see page 180), to serve

1 Mix the flours and baking powder together in a bowl.

2 Rub in the spread and mix in the breadcrumbs, cinnamon, sugar and fruit.

3 Add the egg whites and mix with enough milk to form a soft, dropping consistency.

4 Turn into a 1.2 litre/2 pt/5 cup pudding basin, lightly greased with a very little sunflower oil.

5 Cover with a double thickness of greaseproof (waxed) paper or foil, twisting and folding under the rim to secure.

6 Place on an old saucer in a saucepan with enough boiling water to come halfway up the sides of the basin, or in a steamer over a pan of boiling water, then cover and steam for 2½ hours.

7 Turn out and serve with Low-fat Custard.

Rich and Creamy Brown Rice Pudding

SERVES 4

✴ VERY LOW SATURATED FAT ✴ VERY LOW CHOLESTEROL ✴ HIGH FIBRE

50 g/2 oz/¼ cup brown round-grain rice

450 ml/¾ pt/2 cups water

30 ml/2 tbsp caster (superfine) sugar

420 g/15 oz/1 large can of low-fat evaporated milk

1.5 ml/¼ tsp grated nutmeg

1 Rinse the rice and place in a saucepan with the water. Bring to the boil, reduce the heat and simmer gently for 20 minutes.

2 Stir in the sugar and evaporated milk. Turn into a fairly shallow ovenproof dish.

3 Dust with nutmeg, then place in a preheated oven at 180°C/350°F/gas mark 4 for about 2–2½ hours or until creamy and golden brown and the rice is tender but nutty. Serve warm.

Baked Apples

SERVES 4

★ ALMOST NO SATURATED FAT ★ NO CHOLESTEROL ★ HIGH FIBRE

4 even-sized cooking (tart) apples

60 ml/4 tbsp mixed dried fruit (fruit cake mix)

20 ml/4 tsp clear honey

30 ml/2 tbsp water

Low-fat Custard (see page 180), to serve

1 Cut out the central core from each apple and slit the skin round the centre with the point of a sharp knife to prevent bursting during cooking.

2 Fill with the dried fruit, packing in firmly. Stand the fruit in a baking dish.

3 Put a teaspoon of honey over each apple and add the water to the dish. Bake in a preheated oven at 190°C/375°F/gas mark 5 for about 50 minutes until the fruit is tender. Serve hot with Low-fat Custard.

The Lightest Egg Custard

✳ VERY LOW SATURATED FAT ✳ LOW CHOLESTEROL ✳ NO FIBRE

1 whole egg

2 egg whites

600 ml/1 pt/2½ cups skimmed milk

30 ml/2 tbsp caster (superfine) sugar

A little sunflower or olive oil spread for greasing

A little grated nutmeg

1 Whisk the egg with the egg whites to mix thoroughly.

2 Bring the milk just to the boil, then whisk into the eggs. Stir in the sugar until dissolved.

3 Lightly grease a 900 ml/1½ pt/3¾ cup ovenproof dish. Pour in the custard and dust with nutmeg.

4 Stand the dish in a roasting tin (pan) and add enough hot water to come halfway up the sides of the dish. Bake in a preheated oven at 160°C/325°F/gas mark 3 for about 1 hour until set. Serve warm or cold.

Profiteroles with Hot Chocolate Sauce

SERVES 4

★ LOW SATURATED FAT ★ LOW CHOLESTEROL ★ HIGH FIBRE

65 g/2½ oz/good ½ cup wholemeal flour

25 g/1 oz/2 tbsp sunflower or olive oil spread

150 ml/¼ pt/⅔ cup water

2 egg whites

150 ml/¼ pt/⅔ cup low-fat whipping cream

Finely grated rind of 1 orange (optional)

1 quantity of Hot Chocolate Sauce (see page 183)

1 Sift the flour into a bowl. Add the bran left behind in the sieve (strainer).

2 Put the spread and water in a saucepan and heat until the fat melts.

3 Add the flour all at once and beat with a wooden spoon until the mixture is smooth and leaves the sides of the pan clean.

4 Remove from the heat and cool slightly.

5 Whisk the egg whites until stiff. Beat a little egg white into the paste to soften it, then fold in the remainder with a metal spoon.

6 Put spoonfuls of the mixture well apart on a baking (cookie) sheet, lined with non-stick baking parchment.

7 Bake in a preheated oven at 200°C/400°F/gas mark 6 for 15 minutes, turn them over and bake for a further 10 minutes until crisp and golden. Transfer to a wire rack, make a slit in the side of each to allow the steam to escape and leave to cool.

8 Whip the cream until peaking and add the orange rind, if using. Scoop any remaining soft dough out of each profiterole, then fill with the cream.

9 Pile into dishes and spoon the hot chocolate sauce over.

Light Brûlée

SERVES 4

★ VERY LOW SATURATED FAT ★ LOW CHOLESTEROL ★ NO FIBRE

1 quantity of The Lightest Egg Custard (see page 147)

45 ml/3 tbsp caster (superfine) sugar

1 Prepare the egg custard. When cooked, leave to cool, then chill.

2 Sprinkle the top liberally with the caster sugar to cover completely. Place under a preheated grill (broiler) until the sugar melts and caramelises. Leave until cold, then chill again before serving.

Banana Pudding

SERVES 4

★ VERY LOW SATURATED FAT ★ VERY LOW CHOLESTEROL ★ HIGH FIBRE

50 g/2 oz/¼ cup sunflower or olive oil spread

45 ml/3 tbsp clear honey

1 egg

30 ml/2 tbsp skimmed milk

30 ml/2 tbsp sultanas (golden raisins)

2 bananas, thickly sliced

75 g/3 oz/¾ cup self-raising (self-rising) wholemeal flour

5 ml/1 tsp baking powder

2.5 ml/½ tsp ground cinnamon

Hot Lemon Sauce (see page 182), to serve

1 Beat the spread and honey together until fluffy.

2 Beat in the egg, milk and sultanas and fold in the bananas.

3 Sift the flour, baking powder and cinnamon over the surface, then sprinkle in the bran left in the sieve (strainer).

4 Fold in lightly with a metal spoon.

5 Wet a 450 g/1 lb loaf tin (pan) and line with non-stick baking parchment. Add the banana mixture and level the surface.

6 Bake in a preheated oven at 180°C/350°F/gas mark 4 for about 40 minutes until risen and golden and a skewer comes out clean when inserted in the centre.

7 Turn out on to a serving dish, remove the paper and serve sliced with Hot Lemon Sauce.

Mulled Claret Jelly

SERVES 6

★ NO SATURATED FAT ★ NO CHOLESTEROL ★ NO FIBRE

450 ml/¾ pt/2 cups claret or other full-bodied red wine

30–45 ml/2–3 tbsp clear honey

1 piece of cinnamon stick

3 cloves

2 lemon slices

1 orange

15 ml/1 tbsp powdered gelatine

1 Put the wine, 30 ml/2 tbsp of the honey, the cinnamon stick, cloves and lemon slices in a saucepan.

2 Squeeze the juice from the orange into a measuring jug and make up to 150 ml/¼ pt/⅔ cup with water. Add the orange shells to the wine.

3 Sprinkle the gelatine over the orange juice mixture in the measuring jug and leave to soften for 5 minutes.

4 Meanwhile, bring the wine to the boil, reduce the heat and simmer gently for 5 minutes. Remove from the heat.

5 Tip the softened gelatine mixture into the wine and stir until completely dissolved.

6 Strain into a 600 ml/1 pt/2½ cup wetted mould or pour into an attractive glass dish. Leave until cold, then chill until set.

7 If using a mould, dip it briefly in hot water, then turn out on to a serving dish. Serve completely plain.

Strawberry Cheese Baskets

SERVES 6

★ VERY LOW SATURATED FAT ★ VERY LOW CHOLESTEROL ★ LOW FIBRE

3 sheets of filo pastry (paste)

25 g/1 oz/2 tbsp sunflower or olive oil spread, melted

100 g/4 oz/½ cup strawberry-flavoured low-fat fromage frais

100 g/4 oz small ripe strawberries, hulled

30 ml/2 tbsp redcurrant jelly (clear conserve)

15 ml/1 tbsp water

1 Lay a sheet of pastry on a board and brush very lightly with the melted spread.

2 Fold in half, then half again and brush again. Cut the rectangle into two squares. Repeat with the remaining pastry.

3 Carefully press into six individual flan tins (pie pans).

4 Brush with the remaining spread.

5 Bake in a preheated oven at 190°C/375°F/gas mark 5 for 15 minutes until crisp and golden. Transfer to a wire rack and leave to cool.

6 Fill with fromage frais and top with the strawberries.

7 Melt the redcurrant jelly with the water. Brush all over the strawberries to glaze. Serve within 1 hour.

Mocha Mousse

SERVES 4

★ VERY LOW SATURATED FAT ★ VERY LOW CHOLESTEROL ★ NO FIBRE

10 ml/2 tsp powdered gelatine

150 ml/¼ pt/⅔ cup hot black coffee

*50 g/2 oz/½ cup low-fat drinking
(sweetened) chocolate powder*

30 ml/2 tbsp caster (superfine) sugar

*420 g/15 oz/1 large can of low-fat
evaporated milk, well chilled*

A little extra chocolate powder for dusting

1 Sprinkle the gelatine over the hot coffee. Stir until completely dissolved.

2 Stir in the drinking chocolate and sugar until dissolved. Leave until cold, then chill until the consistency of egg white.

3 Whisk the evaporated milk until really thick and fluffy.

4 Whisk in the coffee and chocolate mixture. Turn into four serving dishes and chill until set.

5 Dust with a little extra chocolate powder before serving.

Honeyed Kiwis and Oranges

SERVES 6

★ ALMOST NO SATURATED FAT ★ NO CHOLESTEROL ★ SOME FIBRE

4 oranges

45 ml/3 tbsp clear honey

45 ml/3 tbsp water

300 ml/½ pt/1¼ cups apple juice

4 kiwi fruit

1 Over a saucepan, pare off all the rind from the oranges. Put the rind in the saucepan. Slice the fruit and place in a glass bowl.

2 Add the honey and water to the saucepan. Bring to the boil and boil for 2 minutes.

3 Remove from the heat and stir in the apple juice. Leave until cold, then strain over the oranges.

4 Peel and slice the kiwi fruit and add to the oranges. Stir gently, then chill until very cold.

Apricot-stuffed Pancakes

SERVES 6

★ VERY LOW SATURATED FAT ★ VERY LOW CHOLESTEROL ★ HIGH FIBRE

*1 quantity of Oat Bran and Wholemeal Pancakes
(see page 162)*

*410 g/14 oz/1 large can of apricot halves
in natural juice*

10 ml/2 tsp arrowroot

15 ml/1 tbsp apricot brandy (optional)

*100 g/4 oz/½ cup low-fat plain or
apricot-flavoured fromage frais*

30 ml/2 tbsp toasted flaked (slivered) almonds

1 Make the pancakes and leave to cool.

2 Strain the juice from the apricots into a saucepan. Chop the fruit.

3 Blend the arrowroot into the juice and add the brandy, if using. Bring to the boil, stirring until thickened and clear. Remove from the heat and leave to cool.

4 Stir in the chopped fruit.

5 Spread each pancake with a little fromage frais. Fold into quarters to make a cone shape. Place two on each serving plate. Gently lift up the top flap of each pancake and spoon in the apricot mixture.

6 Scatter the almonds over before serving.

Tropical Fruit Salad

★ ALMOST NO SATURATED FAT ★ NO CHOLESTEROL ★ FAIRLY HIGH FIBRE

300 ml/½ pt/1¼ cups apple juice

1 ripe mango

1 passion fruit

1 small fresh pineapple

2 star fruit

2 kiwi fruit

1 pomegranate

1 Pour the juice into a plastic container with a lid.

2 Peel the mango, mark into small cubes, cutting right through to the stone (pit). Cut the flesh off the stone.

3 Halve the passion fruit and scoop the seeds into the container.

4 Cut the green top off the pineapple, then cut off all the peel. Cut the pineapple into slices, remove any hard core and cut into chunks. Add to the container.

5 Wipe and slice the star fruit, so you have star-shaped slices. Add to the container.

6 Peel and slice the kiwi fruit.

7 Quarter the pomegranate. Bend back the skin, then carefully loosen the juicy seeds and add to the container. Discard any white pith. Cover the container and chill for at least 1 hour to allow the flavours to develop fully. Turn into a glass serving dish and serve very cold.

Melon with Minted Raspberry Drizzle

SERVES 4

⋆ ALMOST NO SATURATED FAT ⋆ NO CHOLESTEROL ⋆ LOW FIBRE

1 honeydew melon

320 g/12 oz/1 medium can of raspberries in natural juice

15 ml/1 tbsp chopped mint

A few small sprigs of mint, to decorate

1 Cut the melon into eight wedges. Scoop out the seeds, then cut off the rind. Cover and chill.

2 Drain off the juice from the raspberries, then purée the fruit in a blender or food processor with the chopped mint. Pass the purée through a sieve (strainer) into a measuring jug. Thin with enough of the juice to form a smooth, pouring consistency. Chill until ready to serve.

3 Lay the melon on serving plates. Drizzle the raspberry sauce over the centres of the melon wedges and decorate each with a small sprig of mint.

Poached Pears in Cider

SERVES 4

★ VERY LOW SATURATED FAT ★ NO CHOLESTEROL ★ FAIRLY HIGH FIBRE

4 ripe dessert pears

15 ml/1 tbsp chopped mixed nuts

15 ml/1 tbsp fresh wholemeal breadcrumbs

10 ml/2 tsp clear honey

300 ml/½ pt/1¼ cups medium cider

1 clove

4 angelica 'leaves' to decorate

1 Peel the pears and cut out a cone-shaped core at the base of each.

2 Mix the nuts with the breadcrumbs and honey and press firmly into the holes.

3 Stand the pears in a casserole dish (Dutch oven) and pour the cider over. Add the clove.

4 Cover and cook in a preheated oven at 160°C/325°F/gas mark 3 for 45 minutes, basting occasionally.

5 Remove from the oven and leave to cool. Chill until ready to serve.

6 Carefully transfer the fruit to four serving dishes. Spoon the syrup around and press an angelica 'leaf' into the top of each.

BREADS, BISCUITS, CAKES AND NIBBLES

The problem with most commercial bakes is they are often high in saturated fat – just what you don't want. Although there are now quite a few ranges of very low-fat biscuits and cakes on the market and it's fine to eat ordinary wholemeal and whole grain breads, there is something very satisfying about having a baking session at home – and even more so when you know they're good for you!

Granary Bread Sticks

MAKES 24

★ VERY LOW SATURATED FAT ★ NO CHOLESTEROL ★ HIGH FIBRE

300 ml/½ pt/1¼ cups skimmed milk

15 ml/1 tbsp olive oil

450 g/1 lb/4 cups granary flour

A pinch of salt

10 ml/2 tsp easy-blend dried yeast

A little hot water

1 Warm the milk and oil until hand-hot.

2 Meanwhile, mix the flour, salt and yeast in a bowl. Add the hot milk mixture and mix, adding a little hot water if necessary, to form a soft but not sticky dough.

3 Knead on a lightly floured surface for about 5 minutes until elastic. Return to the bowl, cover with clingfilm (plastic wrap) and leave in a warm place for about 45 minutes until doubled in bulk.

4 Re-knead and divide into 24 pieces. Roll each piece into a sausage about 30 cm/12 in long. Place on a non-stick baking (cookie) sheet. Leave for 20 minutes to rise again.

5 Bake in a preheated oven at 220°C/425°F/gas mark 7 for about 30 minutes until crisp and brown. Transfer to a wire rack. Leave until cold, then store in an airtight container.

Oat Tortillas

MAKES 12

★ VERY LOW SATURATED FAT ★ NO CHOLESTEROL ★ HIGH FIBRE

100 g/4 oz/1 cup medium oatmeal

100 g/4 oz/1 cup plain (all-purpose) flour

A pinch of salt

5 ml/1 tsp baking powder

250 ml/8 fl oz/1 cup hand-hot water

1 Mix the oatmeal, flour, salt and baking powder in a bowl.

2 Mix in enough of the hot water to form a soft but not sticky dough. Knead gently on a lightly floured surface.

3 Divide into 12 balls and roll out each one on a surface dusted with a mixture of oatmeal and flour.

4 Heat a heavy non-stick frying pan (skillet) until very hot. Cook each tortilla for 1–2 minutes on each side until just browning in patches. Slide out on to a plate and repeat until all the tortillas are cooked. Either keep warm, wrapped in a napkin on a plate over a pan of hot water, or reheat briefly in the microwave when ready to serve.

Oat Bran and Wholemeal Pancakes

MAKES 12

★ VERY LOW SATURATED FAT ★ VERY LOW CHOLESTEROL ★ HIGH FIBRE

Use these for the stuffed pancake recipes given in this book or simply drizzle with warm clear honey and freshly squeezed lemon juice for a delicious pud.

25 g/1 oz/¼ cup oat bran

75 g/3 oz/¾ cup wholemeal flour

A pinch of salt

1 egg

150 ml/¼ pt/⅔ cup skimmed milk

175 ml/6 fl oz/¾ cup water

30 ml/2 tbsp sunflower oil

1 Mix the oat bran and flour in a bowl with the salt.

2 Make a well in the centre and add the egg.

3 Add half the milk and water and half the oil and whisk thoroughly until smooth.

4 Stir in the remaining milk and water. Leave to stand for 30 minutes, if possible.

5 Brush a small non-stick frying pan (skillet) lightly with a little of the remaining oil and heat the pan until your hand feels very hot when held 5 cm/2 in above the pan.

6 Pour 2–3 tbsp/30–45 ml of the batter into the pan and swirl round to coat the base (don't make the pancake too thick). Cook over a fairly high heat until browned underneath and set on top. Flip over and cook the other side.

7 Slide out on to a plate standing over a pan of hot water to keep warm.

8 Repeat steps 6 and 7 until all the batter is used.

Garlic and Herb Bread

SERVES 6

★ VERY LOW SATURATED FAT ★ VERY LOW CHOLESTEROL ★ HIGH FIBRE

1 small wholemeal baguette

50 g/2 oz/¼ cup sunflower or olive oil spread

1–2 garlic cloves, crushed

15 ml/1 tbsp chopped parsley

15 ml/1 tbsp chopped tarragon

1 Cut the bread into 12 slices, not quite through the base crust.

2 Mash the spread with the garlic and herbs. Spread generously between each slice and spread any remainder over the top.

3 Wrap in foil and bake in a preheated oven at 200°C/400°F/gas mark 6 for about 15 minutes until the crust feels crisp and the centre soft when squeezed.

Oat Bran and Sesame Pitta Breads

MAKES 8

★ VERY LOW SATURATED FAT ★ NO CHOLESTEROL ★ HIGH FIBRE

These are delicious filled with tuna or chopped chicken and salad for lunch or cut into fingers and served with a Greek-style dip, such as Minted Yoghurt and Cucumber (see page 179).

225 g/8 oz/2 cups plain (all-purpose) flour, plus extra for dusting

100 g/4 oz/1 cup oat bran

10 ml/2 tsp easy-blend dried yeast

A pinch of salt

60 ml/4 tbsp sunflower oil

175 ml/6 fl oz/¾ cup hand-hot water

45 ml/3 tbsp sesame seeds

1 Mix the flour, oat bran, yeast and salt in a bowl.

2 Add the oil and beat in the hand-hot water to form a soft, slightly sticky dough.

3 Turn out on to a board, well-dusted with flour, and knead for about 5 minutes until smooth and elastic. Alternatively, place the dry ingredients in a food processor and run the machine while adding the water. Continue to run the machine for 1 minute after the dough is formed.

4 Put the dough into a floured bowl, cover with clingfilm (plastic wrap) and leave in a warm place for about 40 minutes until doubled in size.

5 Re-knead the dough and divide into eight pieces.

6 Shape each piece into an oval. Dust a work surface with some sesame seeds and roll out each piece to an flat oval shape. Lift, scatter more sesame seeds on the board, turn over and flatten again slightly to allow the sesame seeds to stick to the dough. If not ready to cook, wrap in clingfilm.

7 Preheat the oven and a baking (cookie) sheet to 230°C/450°F/gas mark 8. Lay four pittas on the hot baking sheet and bake for 3 minutes. Turn over and bake the other sides for a further 3 minutes until just cooked through. Wrap the pittas in a clean cloth while cooking the remainder. Reheat the baking sheet for a few minutes between each batch of baking.

8 To form pockets, split along one edge of each bread with a sharp knife, or cut the breads in half widthways and open each one along the cut. These are best eaten fresh.

Poppy Seed Scones

MAKES 8

★ VERY LOW SATURATED FAT ★ VERY LOW CHOLESTEROL ★ HIGH FIBRE

*100 g/4 oz/1 cup wholemeal self-raising
(self-rising) flour*

100 g/4 oz/1 cup white self-raising flour

5 ml/1 tsp baking powder

50 g/2 oz/¼ cup sunflower or olive oil spread

15 ml/1 tbsp caster (superfine) sugar

30 ml/2 tbsp poppy seeds

90 ml/6 tbsp skimmed milk

5 ml/1 tsp lemon juice

A little extra milk for brushing

*A little sunflower or olive oil spread and
reduced-sugar jam (conserve), to serve*

1 Sift the flours and baking powder into a bowl. Stir in the bran from the sieve (strainer).

2 Rub in the spread, then stir in the sugar and seeds.

3 Mix the milk and lemon juice together and stir into the mixture to form a soft but not sticky dough.

4 Knead gently on a lightly floured surface. Pat out to about 2 cm/¾ in thick and cut into rounds using a 4 cm/1½ in fluted cutter. Re-knead the trimmings and use to make more scones (biscuits).

5 Place well apart on a non-stick baking (cookie) sheet.

6 Brush with a little milk, then bake in a preheated oven at 220°C/425°F/gas mark 7 for 10–12 minutes until risen and golden. Serve split with a scraping of sunflower or olive oil spread and reduced-sugar jam.

Walnut Cheese Loaf

SERVES 4–6

★ VERY LOW SATURATED FAT ★ VERY LOW CHOLESTEROL ★ HIGH FIBRE

1 small wholemeal baguette

50 g/2 oz/¼ cup low-fat soft cheese

25 g/1 oz/2 tbsp sunflower or olive oil spread

15 ml/1 tbsp finely chopped walnuts

15 ml/1 tbsp chopped parsley

1　Cut the bread into 12 slices, not quite through the base crust.

2　Mash the cheese and spread with the walnuts and parsley. Spread between the slices.

3　Wrap in foil and bake in a preheated oven at 200°C/400°F/gas mark 6 for about 15 minutes until the crust feels crisp when squeezed.

Almond Shortbread Slices

★ VERY LOW SATURATED FAT ★ VERY LOW CHOLESTEROL ★ HIGH FIBRE

100 g/4 oz/½ cup sunflower or olive oil spread

50 g/2 oz/¼ cup caster (superfine) sugar

50 g/2 oz/½ cup plain (all-purpose) flour

50 g/2 oz/½ cup wholemeal flour

75 g/3 oz/¾ cup ground almonds

A few drops of natural almond essence (extract)

A little sunflower oil for greasing

1 Beat the spread and sugar together until light and fluffy.

2 Work in the remaining ingredients to form a soft dough.

3 Press into a lightly oiled 18 × 28 cm/7 × 11 in Swiss roll tin (jelly roll pan). Prick all over with a fork.

4 Bake in a preheated oven at 160°C/325°F/gas mark 3 for about 40 minutes until a pale golden brown.

5 Mark into wide fingers with a knife, then leave until completely cold before removing from the tin. Store in an airtight container.

Hazelnut Macaroons

MAKES 10

★ VERY LOW SATURATED FAT ★ NO CHOLESTEROL ★ SOME FIBRE

You can use ground almonds and almond essence (extract) instead, if you prefer.

1 egg white

75 g/3 oz/¾ cup ground hazelnuts (filberts)

75 g/3 oz/⅓ cup caster (superfine) sugar

15 ml/1 tbsp ground rice

1.5 ml/¼ tsp vanilla essence

10 whole blanched hazelnuts

1 Line a non-stick baking (cookie) sheet with rice paper.

2 Whisk the egg white until very frothy but not stiff.

3 Beat in the hazelnuts, sugar, ground rice and vanilla essence.

4 Spoon ten mounds of the mixture well apart on the rice paper. Top each with a whole hazelnut.

5 Bake in a preheated oven at 160°C/325°F/gas mark 3 for about 25 minutes until pale golden brown. Leave to cool. Carefully cut round each one with scissors. Store in an airtight container.

Raspberry Angel Cake

SERVES 6–8

★ ALMOST NO SATURATED FAT ★ NO CHOLESTEROL ★ LOW FIBRE

50 g/2 oz/½ cup plain (all-purpose) flour

100 g/4 oz/½ cup caster (superfine) sugar

4 egg whites

2.5 ml/½ tsp cream of tartar

2.5 ml/½ tsp vanilla essence (extract)

45 ml/3 tbsp reduced-sugar raspberry jam (conserve)

5 ml/1 tsp icing (confectioners') sugar, sifted

1 Sift the flour twice. Sift the caster sugar to make sure there are no lumps at all.

2 Whisk the egg whites until white but not stiff. Stir in the cream of tartar, then whisk until stiff and glossy.

3 Lightly whisk in the sugar and vanilla.

4 Sprinkle the flour over and fold in very gently with a metal spoon.

5 Turn into a deep 18 cm/7 in round cake tin (pan); do not grease the tin.

6 Bake in a preheated oven at 140°C/275°F/gas mark 1 for 30 minutes. Turn the heat up to 160°C/325°F/gas mark 3 and cook for a further 40 minutes until risen and golden and the centre springs back when lightly pressed.

7 Cool slightly, then turn out on to a wire rack to cool.

8 When cold, split in half, fill with the jam, then dust the top with the icing sugar.

Chocolate Angel Cake Deluxe

SERVES 6–8

★ VERY LOW SATURATED FAT ★ VERY LOW CHOLESTEROL ★ LOW FIBRE

Prepare as for Raspberry Angel Cake (see page 170), but use half reduced-fat drinking (sweetened) chocolate powder and half plain flour. Fill with 45 ml/3 tbsp chocolate-flavoured low-fat fromage frais before dusting with icing (confectioners') sugar.

Speciality Flapjacks

MAKES 18

★ VERY LOW SATURATED FAT ★ VERY LOW CHOLESTEROL ★ HIGH FIBRE

75 g/3 oz/⅓ cup sunflower or olive oil spread

25 g/1 oz/2 tbsp light brown sugar

30 ml/2 tbsp clear honey

175 g/6 oz/1½ cups Original Oat Crunch cereal

50 g/2 oz/½ cup plain (all-purpose) flour

1 Melt the spread, sugar and honey in a saucepan.

2 Stir in the remaining ingredients until well mixed.

3 Turn into a non-stick 18 cm/7 in square baking tin (pan) and press down well.

4 Bake in a preheated oven at 190°C/375°F/gas mark 5 for about 12 minutes or until golden. Cool slightly, then mark into 18 fingers. Leave until completely cold before removing from the tin. Store in an airtight container.

Date and Walnut Loaf

MAKES 1 LOAF

★ VERY LOW SATURATED FAT ★ VERY LOW CHOLESTEROL ★ HIGH FIBRE

225 g/8 oz/2 cups wholemeal self-raising (self-rising) flour

225 g/8 oz/2 cups white self-raising flour

25 g/1 oz/2 tbsp sunflower or olive oil spread

45 ml/3 tbsp clear honey

75 g/3 oz/½ cup chopped stoned (pitted) dates

75 g/3 oz/¾ cup walnuts, chopped

375 ml/13 fl oz/1½ cups skimmed milk

5 ml/1 tsp bicarbonate of soda (baking soda)

A little sunflower or olive oil spread, to serve

1 Mix the two flours together in a large bowl.

2 Rub in the spread.

3 Stir in the honey, dates and nuts.

4 Mix a little of the milk with the bicarbonate of soda and add to the bowl with enough of the remaining milk to form a soft dough.

5 Turn into a non-stick 900 g/2 lb loaf tin (pan), base-lined with non-stick baking parchment.

6 Bake in a preheated oven at 190°C/375°F/gas mark 5 for about 1 hour or until risen and golden and a skewer inserted in the centre comes out clean.

7 Cool slightly, then turn out on to a wire rack, remove the paper and leave to cool. Serve sliced and spread with a scraping of sunflower or olive oil spread.

Microwave Dry-roasted Nuts

★ VERY LOW SATURATED FAT ★ NO CHOLESTEROL ★ HIGH FIBRE

*Peanuts are cheapest, but I love a mixture of almonds,
hazelnuts and cashews.*

Put 45 ml/3 tbsp raw, shelled peanuts (or other nuts) in a
ring on a piece of kitchen paper (paper towel) on a plate.
Microwave on High for 3–4 minutes, stirring once or
twice, until browned. Cool and repeat with as many nuts
as you like. Store in an airtight container.

Note: If you don't have a microwave, you can cook a
single layer of nuts in a heavy-based non-stick frying pan
(skillet), tossing them over a moderate heat until golden.
Remove from the pan as soon as they are brown or they
will continue cooking and may burn.

Hot Spicy Nuts

Prepare as for the plain dry-roasted nuts (above), but
sprinkle with a few drops of reduced-salt soy sauce, before
cooking. Then, as soon as they are cooked, sprinkle them
with equal quantities of chilli powder and mixed (apple-
pie) spice and toss well before cooling and storing.

Garam Garbanzos

SERVES 4–6

✻ ALMOST NO SATURATED FAT ✻ NO CHOLESTEROL ✻ HIGH FIBRE

425 g/15 oz/1 large can of chick peas (garbanzos),
well drained

15 ml/1 tbsp garam masala

A pinch of salt

1 Dry the chick peas on kitchen paper (paper towels).

2 Spread on a non-stick baking (cookie) sheet. Mix the garam masala with the salt, sprinkle over and toss to coat thoroughly.

3 Bake in a preheated oven at 180°C/350°F/gas mark 4 for about 50 minutes until the chick peas are brown and crunchy. Cool, then store in an airtight tin.

Crispy Potato Skins

Place scrubbed potato peelings in a single layer on a baking (cookie) sheet and sprinkle very lightly with salt. Bake at the top of a preheated oven at 200°C/400°F/gas mark 6 for about 20 minutes or until crisp and golden. Cool, then store in an airtight container.

SAUCES AND DRESSINGS

These are the extras that can lift meals from the mundane to the magnificent: a simple dressing drizzled over a salad, a luscious custard poured over a pie or a smooth savoury sauce, moistening fresh colourful vegetables or a simple grilled chicken breast. But they are often full of saturated fat in the form of cream or butter, which is not what you want. These recipes, however, are all very low in saturated fat and are as delicious as any I've ever tasted.

Simple Low-fat White Sauce

SERVES 4

★ ALMOST NO SATURATED FAT ★ VERY LOW CHOLESTEROL ★ LOW FIBRE

45 ml/3 tbsp plain (all-purpose) flour

300 ml/½ pt/1¼ cups skimmed milk

A small knob of sunflower or olive oil spread

1 bouquet garni sachet

A pinch of salt

Freshly ground black or white pepper

1 Put the flour in a saucepan and gradually whisk in the milk.

2 Add the spread and bouquet garni sachet.

3 Bring to the boil and cook for 2 minutes, stirring all the time until thickened and smooth.

4 Squeeze the bouquet garni sachet against the side of the pan to extract the maximum flavour, then discard. Season the sauce to taste with salt and pepper. Use as required.

Variations

Parsley Sauce
Prepare as for Simple Low-fat White Sauce (above) but add 30 ml/2 tbsp chopped parsley to the sauce once cooked.

Cheese Sauce
Prepare as for Simple Low-fat White Sauce (above) but grate 50 g/2 oz/½ cup strong low-fat Cheddar cheese and add after removing the bouquet garni.

Mushroom Sauce

Stew 4–5 finely chopped button mushrooms in 30 ml/ 2 tbsp water in a covered pan for 3 minutes. Remove the lid and boil rapidly, if necessary, to evaporate any remaining liquid. Stir into a quantity of Simple Low-fat White Sauce and add a squeeze of lemon juice, if liked.

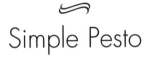

Simple Pesto

SERVES 4

★ VERY LOW SATURATED FAT ★ VERY LOW CHOLESTEROL ★ SOME FIBRE

Add to cooked wholemeal pasta and toss over a gentle heat before serving, spread on slices of ciabatta bread and grill until melted, or use as a stuffing for chicken breasts or fish.

20 basil leaves

1 large sprig of parsley

50 g/2 oz/½ cup pine nuts

1 large garlic clove, halved

45 ml/3 tbsp olive oil

30 ml/2 tbsp grated Parmesan cheese

A pinch of salt

Freshly ground black pepper

1 Put the herbs, nuts and garlic in a blender or food processor. Run the machine briefly to chop.

2 Gradually add the oil, with the machine running, to form a thick paste. Stop the machine and scrape down the sides a few times.

3 Add the cheese and some pepper and run the machine again to form a glistening paste. Store in a screw-topped jar in the fridge for up to 2 weeks.

Red Almond Pesto

SERVES 4

★ VERY LOW SATURATED FAT ★ VERY LOW CHOLESTEROL ★ SOME FIBRE

Use as for Simple Pesto (see page 177).

1 large garlic clove, halved

50 g/2 oz/½ cup ground almonds

15 basil leaves

4 sun-dried tomatoes in olive oil, drained, reserving the oil

30 ml/2 tbsp grated Parmesan cheese

30 ml/2 tbsp hot water

A pinch of salt

Freshly ground black pepper

1 Put the garlic, almonds, basil and tomatoes in a blender or food processor and run the machine briefly to chop.

2 Gradually add 30 ml/2 tbsp of the reserved oil, with the machine running, to form a thick paste. Stop the machine and scrape down the sides a few times.

3 Add the cheese, water and some pepper. Run the machine again to form a paste. Store in a screw-topped jar in the fridge for up to 2 weeks.

Minted Yoghurt and Cucumber

SERVES 4

★ VERY LOW SATURATED FAT ★ VERY LOW CHOLESTEROL ★ LOW FIBRE

*Use this as a dip with Oat Bran and Sesame Pitta Breads
(see page 160), to top jacket baked potatoes or to serve
with curries.*

5 cm/2 in piece of cucumber, grated

5 ml/1 tsp dried mint

1 small garlic clove, crushed (optional)

150 ml/¼ pt/⅔ cup low-fat plain yoghurt

Freshly ground black pepper

1 Squeeze the grated cucumber to remove excess moisture. Place in a bowl.

2 Add the remaining ingredients and mix thoroughly. Chill until ready to serve.

Low-fat Custard

SERVES 4

★ ALMOST NO SATURATED FAT ★ VERY LOW CHOLESTEROL ★ NO FIBRE

45 ml/3 tbsp cornflour (cornstarch)

300 ml/½ pt/1¼ cups skimmed milk

5 ml/1 tsp vanilla essence (extract)

15 ml/1 tbsp caster (superfine) sugar

A few drops of yellow food colouring (optional)

1 Blend the cornflour with a little of the milk in a saucepan.

2 Stir in the remaining milk, the vanilla essence and sugar.

3 Bring to the boil and cook for 2 minutes, stirring all the time, until thickened and smooth. Colour with a few drops of food colouring, if liked.

Chocolate Custard

SERVES 4

★ VERY LOW SATURATED FAT ★ VERY LOW CHOLESTEROL ★ NO FIBRE

30 ml/2 tbsp reduced-fat drinking (sweetened) chocolate powder

30 ml/2 tbsp cornflour (cornstarch)

300 ml/½ pt/1¼ cups skimmed milk

15 ml/1 tbsp clear honey

1 Blend the chocolate and cornflour with some of the milk in a saucepan.

2 Stir in the remaining milk and add the honey.

3 Bring to the boil and cook for 2 minutes, stirring all the time, until thickened and smooth. Serve hot.

Hot Lemon Sauce

SERVES 4

★ ALMOST NO SATURATED FAT ★ ALMOST NO CHOLESTEROL ★ LOW FIBRE

Finely grated rind and juice of 1 large lemon

Water

20 ml/4 tsp cornflour (cornstarch) or arrowroot

5 ml/1 tsp sunflower spread

45 ml/3 tbsp clear honey

1 Make the lemon rind and juice up to 300 ml/½ pt/ 1¼ cups with water.

2 Blend a little with the cornflour or arrowroot in a saucepan, then stir in the remainder. Add the spread.

3 Bring to the boil and cook for 2 minutes, stirring. Sweeten with honey.

Hot Chocolate Sauce

SERVES 4

★ VERY LOW SATURATED FAT ★ VERY LOW CHOLESTEROL ★ NO FIBRE

1 low-calorie chocolate caramel bar

90 ml/6 tbsp skimmed milk

15 g/½ oz/1 tbsp sunflower or olive oil spread

*15 ml/1 tbsp reduced-fat drinking
(sweetened) chocolate powder*

1 Cut the bar into pieces and place in a saucepan.

2 Add the remaining ingredients and heat gently, stirring all the time, until smooth and thickened.

3 Serve hot over profiteroles, ice cream or fruit.

Honey Nut Dressing

SERVES 4

★ VERY LOW SATURATED FAT ★ NO CHOLESTEROL ★ SOME FIBRE

30 ml/2 tbsp clear honey

15 ml/1 tbsp sunflower oil

15 ml/1 tbsp lemon juice

15 ml/1 tbsp water

30 ml/2 tbsp finely chopped mixed nuts

15 ml/1 tbsp chopped parsley

Freshly ground black pepper

Put all the ingredients in a screw-topped jar and shake vigorously until well blended. Use as required.

Extra-light Mayonnaise

SERVES 4

★ VERY LOW SATURATED FAT ★ VERY LOW CHOLESTEROL ★ NO FIBRE

30 ml/2 tbsp reduced-calorie mayonnaise

30 ml/2 tbsp low-fat plain yoghurt

5 ml/1 tsp lemon juice

A pinch of salt

A pinch of white pepper

Mix all the ingredients together and use as required.

Lo-French Dressing

★ VERY LOW SATURATED FAT ★ NO CHOLESTEROL ★ NO FIBRE

15 ml/1 tbsp olive oil

30 ml/2 tbsp red or white wine vinegar

30 ml/2 tbsp water

1.5 ml/¼ tsp Dijon mustard

A pinch of salt

A pinch of caster (superfine) sugar

Freshly ground black pepper

Shake all the ingredients together in a screw-topped jar until well blended. Use as required.

Light Cheese Dressing

★ VERY LOW SATURATED FAT ★ VERY LOW CHOLESTEROL ★ LOW FIBRE

60 ml/4 tbsp low-fat soft cheese

10 ml/2 tsp snipped chives

10 ml/2 tsp chopped parsley

30 ml/2 tbsp skimmed milk

5 ml/1 tsp dried onion granules

Freshly ground black pepper

Whisk all the ingredients together with pepper to taste. Thin with a little more milk, if necessary. Use as required.

Gran's Light Dressing

SERVES 4

★ VERY LOW SATURATED FAT ★ VERY LOW CHOLESTEROL ★ NO FIBRE

15 ml/1 tbsp light brown sugar

30 ml/2 tbsp skimmed milk

30 ml/2 tbsp buttermilk or low-fat crème fraîche

2.5 ml/½ tsp made English mustard

A pinch of salt

Freshly ground black pepper

Malt vinegar, to taste

1 Whisk the sugar, milk, buttermilk or crème fraîche, mustard, salt and lots of pepper together in a small bowl or jug.

2 Whisk in vinegar to taste.

Rosy Dressing

SERVES 4

★ VERY LOW SATURATED FAT ★ VERY LOW CHOLESTEROL ★ NO FIBRE

1 quantity of Extra-light Mayonnaise (see page 182)

10 ml/2 tsp reduced-sugar and -salt tomato ketchup (catsup)

2.5 ml/½ tsp Worcestershire sauce

A few drops of Tabasco sauce

Mix all the ingredients together and use as required.

INDEX